Xuyang Li

Body Matched Antennas for Microwave Medical Applications

Karlsruher Forschungsberichte
aus dem Institut für Hochfrequenztechnik und Elektronik

Herausgeber: Prof. Dr.-Ing. Thomas Zwick

Band 72

Body Matched Antennas for Microwave Medical Applications

by
Xuyang Li

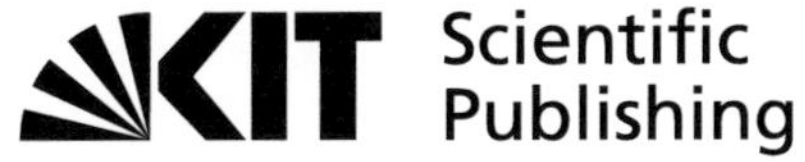

Dissertation, Karlsruher Institut für Technologie (KIT)
Fakultät für Elektrotechnik und Informationstechnik, 2013

Impressum

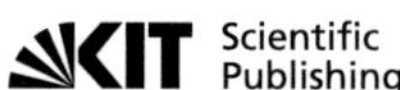 Scientific
Publishing

Karlsruher Institut für Technologie (KIT)
KIT Scientific Publishing
Straße am Forum 2
D-76131 Karlsruhe

KIT Scientific Publishing is a registered trademark of Karlsruhe
Institute of Technology. Reprint using the book cover is not allowed.

www.ksp.kit.edu

Print on Demand 2014

ISSN 1868-4696
ISBN 978-3-7315-0147-3

Editor's Preface

Originally motivated by the ever increasing demand on the high data rate in the field of mobile communication, intensive research has been underway since many years on a new technology: the ultra wideband (UWB) technology. The transmit signal spreads in a huge bandwidth, which results in an extremely low power spectrum density and therefore low interference to other radio communication services. The frequency spectrum released in many parts of the world since some years ago paves the way for the future commercial UWB systems and their research works. Meanwhile, the research focus on applications relevant to UWB has shifted definitively to radar. Of these research works, the medical diagnosis based on UWB technology plays an essential role. Though in general the UWB technology cannot achieve the performance of the existing technologies such as magnetic resonance imaging (MRI), computed tomography (CT scan) and sonography using ultrasound, the imaging systems based on microwaves could well be a complementary method to these existing medical diagnosis systems. On the one hand, the new UWB systems can be considerably much cheaper and more portable than MRT and CT. On the other hand, microwaves have an advantage compared to ultrasound, in that they can penetrate through the bone and "see" the tissues behind it. Besides that, the UWB technology enables wireless data transmission from implantable sensors inside the human body to outside equipment with relatively high data rates. However, all of the medical applications based on UWB technology have a common problem: the relatively high signal attenuation caused by the human tissues. A basic approach to solving this problem is to place the antenna directly on the body. In this way, the strong reflection from the boundary of air and human body can be significantly reduced. Moreover, the approach allows a reduction of the antenna size due to the reduced wavelength, which is not only essential for implanted devices but also for a medical imaging system, since multichannel systems with an antenna array are required.

In his dissertation Mr. Li developed the concepts and basic techniques for the realization of body-matched antennas for medical applications. The major challenges of this work were caused by the fact that these antennas will directly radiate into a medium different from vacuum/air. This does not only lead to different antenna concepts and designs but also does not allow an antenna characterization by the standard antenna measurement setups. Therefore Xuyang Li also had to develop a novel antenna characterization setup for body-matched antennas, and I am positive that his work will attract much interest from the research community worldwide. With his new miniaturization and optimization strategies for ultra-wideband body-matched antennas Mr. Li achieved significant size reductions with concurrent efficiency maximization so I strongly believe that his work will draw attention in the research community worldwide. My personal wish for Mr. Li is that his creativity and great engineering talent together with his organizational skills and team spirit will continue to earn him both scientific and economic success.

Prof. Dr.-Ing. Thomas Zwick
– Director of the IHE –

Forschungsberichte aus dem
Institut für Höchstfrequenztechnik und Elektronik (IHE)
der Universität Karlsruhe (TH) (ISSN 0942-2935)

Herausgeber: Prof. Dr.-Ing. Dr. h.c. Dr.-Ing. E.h. mult. Werner Wiesbeck

Forschungsberichte aus dem
Institut für Höchstfrequenztechnik und Elektronik (IHE)
der Universität Karlsruhe (TH) (ISSN 0942-2935)

Forschungsberichte aus dem
Institut für Höchstfrequenztechnik und Elektronik (IHE)
der Universität Karlsruhe (TH) (ISSN 0942-2935)

Forschungsberichte aus dem
Institut für Höchstfrequenztechnik und Elektronik (IHE)
der Universität Karlsruhe (TH) (ISSN 0942-2935)

Fortführung als
"Karlsruher Forschungsberichte aus dem Institut für Hochfrequenztechnik
und Elektronik" bei KIT Scientific Publishing
(ISSN 1868-4696)

Karlsruher Forschungsberichte aus dem
Institut für Hochfrequenztechnik und Elektronik
(ISSN 1868-4696)

Herausgeber: Prof. Dr.-Ing. Thomas Zwick

Die Bände sind unter www.ksp.kit.edu als PDF frei verfügbar
oder als Druckausgabe bestellbar.

Band 55   Sandra Knörzer
          **Funkkanalmodellierung für OFDM-Kommunikationssysteme
          bei Hochgeschwindigkeitszügen** (2009)
          ISBN 978-3-86644-361-7

Band 56   Thomas Fügen
          **Richtungsaufgelöste Kanalmodellierung und Systemstudien
          für Mehrantennensysteme in urbanen Gebieten** (2009)
          ISBN 978-3-86644-420-1

Band 57   Elena Pancera
          **Strategies for Time Domain Characterization of UWB
          Components and Systems** (2009)
          ISBN 978-3-86644-417-1

Band 58   Jens Timmermann
          **Systemanalyse und Optimierung der Ultrabreitband-
          Übertragung** (2010)
          ISBN 978-3-86644-460-7

Band 59   Juan Pontes
          **Analysis and Design of Multiple Element Antennas
          for Urban Communication** (2010)
          ISBN 978-3-86644-513-0

Band 60   Andreas Lambrecht
          **True-Time-Delay Beamforming für ultrabreitbandige
          Systeme hoher Leistung** (2010)
          ISBN 978-3-86644-522-2

Band 61   Grzegorz Adamiuk
          **Methoden zur Realisierung von dual-orthogonal, linear
          polarisierten Antennen für die UWB-Technik** (2010)
          ISBN 978-3-86644-573-4

Band 62   Jutta Kühn
          **AlGaN/GaN-HEMT Power Amplifiers with Optimized
          Power-Added Efficiency for X-Band Applications** (2011)
          ISBN 978-3-86644-615-1

Karlsruher Forschungsberichte aus dem
Institut für Hochfrequenztechnik und Elektronik
(ISSN 1868-4696)

Band 63 Małgorzata Janson
Hybride Funkkanalmodellierung für ultrabreitbandige
MIMO-Systeme (2011)
ISBN 978-3-86644-639-7

Band 64 Mario Pauli
Dekontaminierung verseuchter Böden durch
Mikrowellenheizung (2011)
ISBN 978-3-86644-696-0

Band 65 Thorsten Kayser
Feldtheoretische Modellierung der Materialprozessierung
mit Mikrowellen im Durchlaufbetrieb (2011)
ISBN 978-3-86644-719-6

Band 66 Christian Andreas Sturm
Gemeinsame Realisierung von Radar-Sensorik und
Funkkommunikation mit OFDM-Signalen (2012)
ISBN 978-3-86644-879-7

Band 67 Huaming Wu
Motion Compensation for Near-Range Synthetic Aperture
Radar Applications (2012)
ISBN 978-3-86644-906-0

Band 68 Friederike Brendel
Millimeter-Wave Radio-over-Fiber Links based on
Mode-Locked Laser Diodes (2013)
ISBN 978-3-86644-986-2

Band 69 Lars Reichardt
Methodik für den Entwurf von kapazitätsoptimierten
Mehrantennensystemen am Fahrzeug (2013)
ISBN 978-3-7315-0047-6

Band 70 Stefan Beer
Methoden und Techniken zur Integration von 122 GHz
Antennen in miniaturisierte Radarsensoren (2013)
ISBN 978-3-7315-0051-3

Band 71 Łukasz Zwirełło
Realization Limits of Impulse-Radio UWB Indoor
Localization Systems (2013)
ISBN 978-3-7315-0114-5

Band 72 Xuyang Li
Body Matched Antennas for Microwave Medical Applications (2014)
ISBN 978-3-7315-0147-3

Body Matched Antennas for Microwave Medical Applications

Zur Erlangung des akademischen Grades eines

DOKTOR-INGENIEURS

von der Fakultät für
Elektrotechnik und Informationstechnik,
am Karlsruher Institut für Technologie (KIT)

genehmigte

DISSERTATION

von

Dipl.-Ing. Xuyang Li

geb. in Zhejiang, China

Tag der mündlichen Prüfung: 28. 05. 2013
Hauptreferent: Prof. Dr.-Ing. Thomas Zwick
Korreferent: Prof. Dr. rer. nat. habil. Matthias Hein

Abstract

The microwave technique is a currently very attractive technique for medical applications. It uses non-ionizing electromagnetic waves and has good penetration capability into human tissues (in the GHz range). Since the ultra wideband (UWB) technology features high resolution imaging and low system complexity, the making of a flexible yet portable device for medical diagnosis can be achieved. Moreover wireless data transmission of physiological and vital signs of patients for monitoring purposes are also feasible due to the high data transmission capability of wideband microwave signals. With these, a new future telemedicine home system can be envisioned, in which the vital signs of the patients can be detected and monitored in real time and hence improving their mobility as well as their quality of life. In these microwave medical systems, it is ultimately the performance of the antennas for radiating and receiving the signals that is the governing factor of the overall system performance.

In this thesis, new concepts of body-matched antennas for microwave medical applications were developed, where the antennas are placed directly on the human body or implanted in the human body. The antenna designs are mainly for microwave medical diagnosis and data telemetry systems. Two types of antennas were designed - *on-body matched antennas* for microwave medical diagnosis and *implantable antennas* for data telemetry. These antennas are designed to be matched to the human body to strongly reduce the reflection at the boundary of air and skin, hence the dielectric properties of different human tissues and complex multiple-layered human body must be taken into account. Challenges of the antenna design with regard to the efficient design process, miniaturization, application specific performance, characterization and verification of the antennas arise and are the main focus as well as contributions of the thesis.

The basis of the antenna design and matching comes from the study of the properties of the different human tissues and the microwave propagation in the human body. Following a systematic antenna design and optimization procedure, the resulting antennas were then further miniaturized for compactness. Since the antennas operate in the near-field, novel measurement verification systems were also designed to measure the radiation performance of the antennas. The resulting set of antennas developed were compact in size yet maintained a high radiation performance. They are found to be suited as implantable antennas for IMDs and as on-body matched antennas for microwave medical imaging, operating at different frequency bands. The applicability of the on-body matched antennas for microwave imaging is also demonstrated by means of a measurement demonstrator system with an antenna array for the detection of hemorrhagic stroke. The results show the high detection capability for stroke due to the low operational frequency, high front-to-back ratio, and the small antenna size. All these contributions enable a portable system to complement the current medical applications with the objective to provide more advanced healthcare systems.

Vorwort

Die vorliegende Arbeit entstand während meiner Zeit als wissenschaftlicher Mitarbeiter am Institut für Hochfrequenztechnik und Elektronik (IHE) des Karlsruher Instituts für Technologie (KIT). Hiermit möchte ich mich herzlich bei allen Personen bedanken, die zum Gelingen dieser Arbeit beigetragen haben.

Mein besonderer Dank gilt meinem Doktorvater, Herrn Prof. Thomas Zwick, für die konstruktiven inhaltlichen Anregungen zu dieser Arbeit und die vielfältige fachliche sowie außerfachliche Unterstützung meiner wissenschaftlichen Tätigkeit. Bedanken möchte ich mich auch bei Herrn Prof. Matthias Hein für die freundliche Übernahme des Korreferats und die zügige Erstellung des Zweitgutachtens. Im Weiteren danke ich Herrn Prof. Werner Wiesbeck herzlich, der meine fachlichen und persönlichen Fähigkeiten stets gefördert hat. Ein Dankeschön an M.Sc. Yoke Leen Sit, Dr.-Ing. Grzegorz Adamiuk, Dr.-Ing. Juan Pontes und Dipl.-Ing. Kai-Philipp Pahl, für ihre sorgfältige Durchsicht und die wertvollen Ratschläge. Ferner möchte ich meinen Zimmerkollegen, allen wissenschaftlichen Mitarbeitern und allen Kollegen aus Verwaltung und Technik meinen Dank aussprechen für die außergewöhnliche Atmosphäre und die hervorragende Zusammenarbeit. Schließlich gilt mein ausdrücklicher Dank meinen Studierenden, die im Rahmen ihrer Abschlussarbeiten mit hohem Engagement und Kreativität einen wichtigen Teil zu meiner Arbeit geleistet haben.

Nicht zuletzt geht mein herzlicher Dank an meine Familie für ihre uneingeschränkte Förderung meines Auslandsstudiums und ihre liebevolle Unterstützung auf dem Weg zu meiner Promotion.

Karlsruhe, im November 2013

Xuyang Li

Contents

Acronyms and Symbols

Acronyms

AUT	Antenna Under Test
BW	Bandwidth
CIR	Channel Impulse Response
Co-pol	Co-polarization
CPW	Coplanar Waveguide
CST	Computer Simulation Technology
CT	Computed Tomography
DAS	Delay and Sum
EM	Electro-Magnetic
E-field	Electric Field
FCC	Federal Communications Commission
FIR	Finite Impulse Response
ICNIRP	International Commission on Non-Ionizing Radiation Protection
IF	Intermediate Frequency
IFFT	Inverse Fast Fourier Transformation
IMDs	Implanted Medical Devices
IR	Impulse-Radio
IR-UWB	Impulse-Radio Ultra Wideband
ISM	Industrial, Scientific and Medical Radio
LNA	Low Noise Amplifier
MAMI	Multistatic Adaptive Microwave Imaging
Matlab	MATrix LABoratory
MedRadio	Medical Device Radio

MICS	Medical Implant Communication Service
MIST	Microwave Imaging via Space-Time
MRI	Magnetic Resonance Imaging
NF-FF	Near-Field to Far-Field
PEG	Polyethylene Glycol
PN	Pseudo-Noise
Radar	Radio Detection and Ranging
RF	Radio Frequency
RFID	Radio-Frequency Identification
SA	Synthetic Aperture
SAR	Specific Absorption Rate
SCR	Signal-to-Clutter Ratio
SNR	Signal-to-Noise Ratio
TEM	Transverse Electromagnetic
UWB	Ultra Wideband
VNA	Vector Network Analyzer
X-pol	Cross-polarization

Symbols

Lower case letters

c_0	speed of light in vacuum ($\approx 2,997925 \cdot 10^8$ m/s)
c_m	speed of light in medium
d	distance
d_p	distortion of pulse
e	Euler's constant (2.718...)
f	frequency
f_H	highest operational frequency
f_L	lowest operational frequency
$h_\mathrm{c}(t)$	channel impulse response
h_s	thickness of substrate
k	wave number

k_{sp}	fraction of the resonant wavelength
r	distance in spherical coordinate
r_{A}	distance to antenna
t	time
$u_{\mathrm{T}}(t)$	transmitted signal in the time domain
$u_{\mathrm{R}}(t)$	received signal in the time domain
$x(t)$	input signal of the beamformer
$y(t)$	output signal of the beamformer
x, y, z	Cartesian coordinate

Capital letters

B	Magnetic flux density
C	Antenna pattern
CF	Coherence factor of the beamformer
C_{i}	Heat capacity of tissues
C_{s}	Circumference of the slot
D	Dielectric flux density
D_{a}	Attenuation
D_{A}	Dimension of antenna
E	Electric field intensity
F	Plane wave spectrum
F_{p}	Fidelity of pulse
F/B	Front-to-back ratio
G	Antenna gain
G_{p}	Antenna peak gain
H	Magnetic field intensity
$H(f)$	Transfer function in the frequency domain
$H_{\mathrm{c}}(f)$	Transfer function of the channel
$H_{\mathrm{Rx}}(f)$	Transfer function of the receiving antenna
$H_{\mathrm{s}}(f)$	Transfer function of the system
$H_{\mathrm{Tx}}(f)$	Transfer function of the transmitting antenna
I	Current

J	Conduction current density
L	Scan length of planar-rectangular near-field measurement
L_{sp}	Effective electrical length of the meandered strips
P_{rad}	Radiated power
R_{ff}	Fraunhofer distance
R_{L}	Loss resistance of an antenna
R_{nf}	Fresnel distance
R_{rad}	Radiation resistance of an antenna
S	Reflection characteristic of the human abdomen model
S_{L}	Power density in lossy medium
S_{11}	Input reflection coefficient at port 1
S_{21}	Forward transmission coefficient from port 1 to port 2
X_{A}	Reactance of an antenna
$X(f)$	Transfer function of a transmitted signal
$Y(f)$	Transfer function of a received signal
Z_{A}	Antenna impedance
Z_{m}	Characteristic wave impedance in medium
Z_0	Characteristic impedance of feed lines (microstrip, slotline, etc.) (50 Ω in this work)
Z_{F0}	Characteristic wave impedance in free space ($\approx 377\,\Omega$)

Greek symbols

α	Attenuation constant
α_n	Distribution parameter in the Cole-Cole equation
β	Phase constant
δ	Loss tangent
δ_{p}	Penetration depth
$\Delta\varepsilon$	Magnitude of the dispersion in the Cole-Cole equation
ΔT	Change in temperature
Δt	Time period
ε	Permittivity
ε_{r}	Relative permittivity

$\varepsilon_{r,eff}$	Effective relative permittivity
ε_∞	Permittivity at $\omega \to \infty$ (highest frequency) in the Debye equation
ε_s	Permittivity at $\omega \to 0$ (lowest frequency) in the Debye equation
ε_0	Permittivity of free space ($8.854 \cdot 10^{-12}$ F/m)
φ	Azimuth angle of spherical coordinate
γ	Complex propagation constant
Γ	Reflection coefficient
η	Radiation efficiency of an antenna
η_p	Penetration efficiency
λ	Wave length
λ_m	Wave length in medium
μ	Permeability
μ_0	Permeability of free space ($4\pi \cdot 10^{-7}$V.s/(A.m))
π	Pi (3.14159...)
θ	Polar angle of spherical coordinate
ρ	Mass density
σ	Conductivity
σ_i	Static ionic conductivity in the Cole-Cole equation
τ	Time delay of signal
τ'	Relaxation time in the Cole-Cole equation
τ_{ij}	Time delay in the beamformer
ω	Angular frequency
ω_{ij}	Beamformer apodization weights

Mathematical notation and symbols

j	Imaginary unit $j = \sqrt{-1}$
s	Variable
$\vec{s}$	Vector
$\underline{s}$	Complex variable
∇	Nabla
$\nabla \cdot \vec{s}$	Divergence of vector field

$\nabla \times \vec{s}$	Rotation of vector field
$\lvert \cdot \rvert$	Absolute value
$\log$	Logarithm
$\tan$	Tangent

1. Introduction

It was in 1840 that the pioneers Recamier and Pravaz experimentally demonstrated the use of the electric current at sub-microwave frequency to generate heat for the destruction of uterine cancer [Guy84]. However, the interest in using microwaves with a short wavelength for medical applications only began in World War II. Hollman proposed the use of microwaves at 1.2 GHz to heat the deep tissues for therapeutic applications in Germany in 1938 [Hol38]. In 1939, Hemingway and Stenstrom reviewed the short-wave diathermy in the United States, which is a method of applying heat using microwaves for therapeutic purposes in medicine [Ste23]. However, the development and clinical trials of these concepts were strictly limited to low frequencies (below 100 MHz) at that time, since the technologies for radio frequency (RF) hardware had not been developed. Today, thanks to the rapid development in semiconductor technology and various signal processing techniques, there is a growing interest in the research and development of medical applications based on microwave techniques.

1.1. State-of-the-art microwave medical applications

So far conventional technologies such as magnetic resonance imaging (MRI) using magnetic fields, mammography and computed tomography (CT scan) using X-ray, sonography using ultrasound are widely used for medical diagnosis (such as cancer, bone imaging, etc.). These technologies provide good sensitivity regarding the image contrast between the different tissues and good spatial resolution in the sub-millimeter range. However, the MRI system is not readily available at all hospitals due to the bulky machinery required, the high manufacturing cost and the relatively long examination time.

Mammography and CT scan, using ionizing radiation, are techniques with intrinsic hazards and increase the risk of cancer incidence. Moreover, the painful examinations associated with mammography have to be tolerated by the patients. The ultrasound technique performs without ionization and is preferred for medical diagnosis. However, it cannot penetrate bones and air due to their strong reflections that cause acoustic shadows [MV98].

Compared to problems and risks associated with these technologies, the microwave technique for medical applications uses non-ionizing electromagnetic waves, which makes it less harmful for the patients compared to mammography and CT scan. Microwaves at low frequencies (below 2 GHz) feature good penetration ability into all human tissues including the bones, in which ultrasound has difficulty to penetrate. A high resolution for microwave medical imaging can be achieved by using wideband microwave signals. Furthermore, microwaves within the same frequency range allow a combination of diagnosis and wireless data transmission, which is not possible using any other technologies for medical applications.

Nowadays, the major microwave applications in the medical field are in data telemetry, medical diagnosis and treatment (see in Figure 1.1). These three applications will be briefly introduced in the following sections.

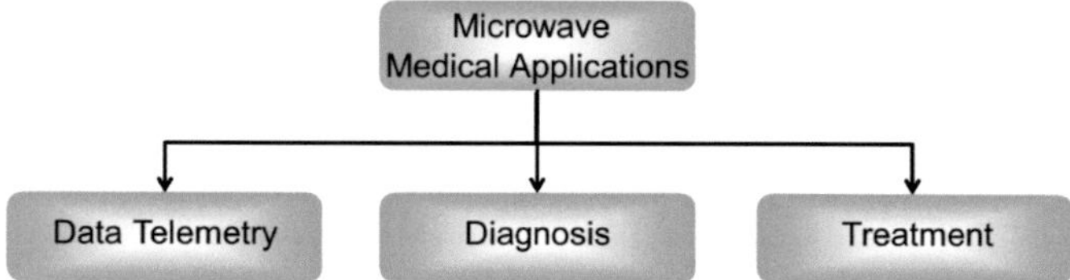

Figure 1.1.: Three major microwave medical applications.

Data telemetry

Data telemetry in this work refers to wireless data transmission using microwaves between implanted medical devices (IMDs) and external devices. Due to the rising quality of life and a growing market for health care products, IMDs have gained much interest for healthcare providers in the recent years. Examples of such devices are implantable cardioverter defibrillators [WDJ$^+$96], bladder stimulators [BSAG$^+$00] and pacemakers [VC09], which are widely used. In the case of the traditional IMDs, the wires used to connect to the devices for the acquisition of diagnosis signals increase the pain and risk of infection in the patients. Therefore, a wireless communication link between implants and external devices is strongly desirable. With the wireless link, the continuous monitoring of the state of implanted devices (e.g. battery state) can also be achieved. The external devices can then act as a controller for the implanted devices.

Potential applications of the data telemetry are such as in glucose monitoring for diabetics, cochlear implants, deep brain stimulation [KHT08, QLD03, TDGL11], etc. For glucose monitoring for diabetics, the glucose level is recorded by an implanted biosensor and transmitted by an implantable antenna to the external devices. In the application of cochlear implants, the audio signal can be transmitted directly by an external antenna attached behind the ear to the receiver in the cochlea (cochlear implant). Other applications using data telemetry such as wireless monitoring of body temperature, blood pressure and heart beat rate are addressed in the literature.

To date, there are no other techniques that are more suitable than the microwave technique for the data telemetry between IMDs and external devices. This is because microwaves enable wireless communication links through the human tissues, which significantly improves the quality of life of the patients compared to the use of traditional IMDs with wires.

Medical diagnosis using microwaves

The applications for medical diagnosis are in the detection of breast cancer, stroke, water accumulation in human body, etc. Among these, one of the most important applications of medical diagnosis is the detection of breast cancer, which is the most prevalent form of cancer among women [FAB$^+$07]. Approximately one million women around the world suffer from breast cancer [MJ13]. Therefore, technologies with high accuracy and sensitivity to detect the presence of tumors are required. An almost pain-free examination with a short examination time and a portable apparatus is especially desirable for the detection of early-stage breast cancer.

Stroke detection is the third leading cause of death in the world and is regarded as a challenging issue in the medical world [RFFea07]. In general, stroke causes the loss of brain functionality due to a disturbance of the blood flow to the brain. It is classified into two major categories of ischemic and hemorrhagic stroke, where both require very different medical treatment (therapies) [Lan09, TP08]. Since the diagnosis and determination of the stroke categories must be done within a few hours, flexible and portable devices that are accessible to the public are strongly in demand.

The spectrum of applications of medical diagnosis is extended to the detection and localization of water accumulations in the human body [1]. This application is crucial for people with diseases such as pulmonary edema due to heart failure [FG95] and urinary incontinence. For example, by monitoring the urine in the human bladder, a permanent catheterization can be avoided and the quality of life of these patients can be significantly improved. Portable and low-cost device is required to enable each patient to be equipped with this apparatus.

Microwave signals provide high potential for the imaging of the breast, the bladder or the brain [KCL$^+$09, ARTN11, GJR10]. This is due to the fact that microwaves feature non-ionizing radiation, high range resolution and high penetration ability, which have been discussed and compared with conventional medical imaging techniques at the beginning of this chapter. Moreover, a low system complexity of the microwave system, which enables the realization of a portable apparatus, is emphasized after reviewing the different medical applications.

Microwave medical diagnosis is based on the concept of observing the scattered signals caused by the dielectric contrast, which is the difference of the dielectric properties between the malignant tissues and the surrounding healthy tissues [FLHS02, LBVVH05]. In microwave medical diagnosis, most researches are focused on two main approaches: radar (Radio Detection and Ranging) imaging and microwave tomography. In radar imaging, wideband antennas for high range resolution are applied for synthetic aperture (SA) based operation or multistatic operation based on fixed array [20] [Nik11, KCL$^+$09]. Microwave tomography is based on the reconstruction of the distribution of the complex permittivity by solving the inverse electromagnetic scattering problem. Recently, the microwave holography in medical near-field imaging has been proposed in [ARNT11], which uses a reference wave and sophisticated holographic reconstruction algorithms.

Medical treatment using microwaves

Medical treatment using microwaves is based on using the heat generated by microwave radiation to increase the local temperature to destroy the abnormal tissues (e.g. malignant tissues). This technique is more sensitive and effective compared to ionizing radiation (i.e. X-ray) and chemical toxins (i.e. Chemotherapy) [Roe99]. The related applications range from hyperthermia in the treatment of breast cancer, transurethral microwave thermotherapy to microwave ablation [Kap96, CBHVV04, SDMS05].

In the framework of this thesis, medical treatment using microwaves will not be considered. The focus of this thesis is on the telemedicine system using microwaves for data telemetry and diagnosis.

1.2. Telemedicine using microwaves and its challenges

Telemedicine for the improvement of the quality of health care for patients was introduced two decades ago. Telemedicine refers to the use of telecommunication for the transmission of health information to deliver clinical healthcare from a distance. In this way, the access to the medical services of patients can significantly be improved.

A vision of the future telemedicine for a healthcare system for nursing home residents using microwaves is illustrated in Figure 1.2. The medical diagnosis system serves to monitor health problems such as stroke for prompt diagnosis and treatment. On the other hand, the data transmission between IMDs and external devices are performed simultaneously. In this way, the combination between medical diagnosis and data telemetry using microwaves contributes very positively to the existing healthcare services. The details of the vision are briefly introduced in the following paragraphs.

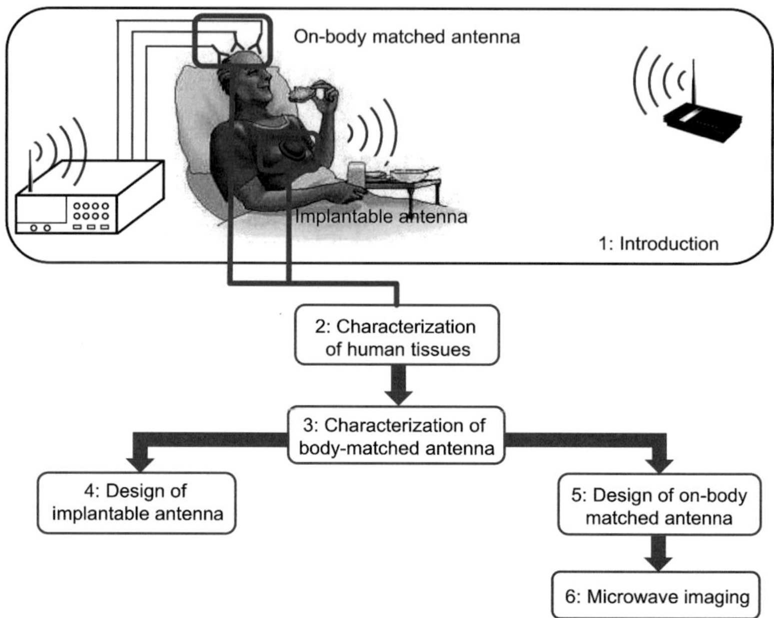

Figure 1.2.: Vision of the telemedicine for nursing home residents using microwaves and the goal as well as organization of the work to realize these applications.

In the data telemetry of this healthcare system, the physiological data (temperature, blood pressure, glucose concentration) or vital signs (such as respiration, heart beating, etc.) are monitored by sensors integrated on the implants. The implants are wirelessly powered by an antenna at a certain frequency (usually very low frequency in the MHz range). The wireless data transmission between implants and external medical devices is performed at a high frequency (in the GHz range). However, the wireless transmission system is normally in low-power stand-by modus and can be awaken by an external signal for operating data transfer at full power at the frequency band licensed for medical devices. At the medical center, the received data is forwarded to the healthcare practitioner to evaluate the patient's status. In the case where abnormalities are detected, the doctor is immediately informed so that necessary actions can be initiated in time.

Simultaneously, as shown in Figure 1.2, medical diagnosis of stroke using microwaves can be performed flexibly and monitored frequently. This diagnosis functions as a complementary method in home healthcare systems compared to traditional technologies (i.e. MRI and CT scan), which can only be performed in hospital due to the bulky devices and high cost. The low system complexity of microwave imaging system enables a flexible and even portable diagnostic device. This system also features a low interference to other microwave systems due to the low regulated radiation power in the respective frequency bands [Com01]. With the help of further image processing, the diagnosis can be evaluated and wirelessly transmitted to the medical center.

However, several technical difficulties in the proposed telemedicine system using microwaves must be overcome, which will be described in the following paragraphs.

From the system point of view, the challenges of wireless data transmission between the implants and external devices are for example low-power consumption, which is critical for the lifespan of the implanted devices. Moreover, wireless data transmission can be strongly limited by radiation regulations in terms of radiation power and operational frequency range. Further challenges are such as robustness against the movement and position of the patients as well as secure and reliable communication [NMdS+07, SCK07].

For microwave medical diagnosis, the signal-to-noise ratio (SNR) of the received signal is a major issue. Since the reflections from the targets (e.g. tumors) are very weak due to the high signal attenuation in human tissues in the GHz range, the SNR of the whole system is thus very low. Therefore, more energy is required to penetrate into human tissues.

With these requirements in mind, one of the main obstacles towards the realization of the vision shown in Figure 1.2 is the development of suitable antennas for IMDs and medical diagnosis using radar imaging. For such applications, the antennas for radiating and receiving the signals is the governing factor of the SNR of the overall system.

In this work, two types of antennas for the purpose of medical applications are considered. They are **implantable antennas** and **on-body matched an-**

tennas. The implantable antennas are used for the data transmission between IMDs and external devices, while the on-body matched antennas are used in diagnosis applications (such as cancer, brain diseases, etc.).

For wireless data transmission of IMDs with external devices, the implantable antennas are located together with IMDs in the human body and surrounded by different human tissues depending on the applications (refer to skin, fat, muscle, etc.).

Different from the on-body matched antenna, antennas can be built for microwave medical diagnosis, which are placed at a distance from the body (termed as **off-body antenna**). In the case of off-body antenna, a strong reflection of the incident waves on the air-skin interface occurs and more than 50% of the energy is back scattered, since the relative permittivity of skin is very large (around 40 at 1 GHz) compared to free space. Furthermore, the distance between antenna and human body introduces additional free space attenuation. Therefore, the energy penetrating into the human body is lower than 10% of the total energy of the incident waves. Moreover, the reflections from the air-skin interface are dominant, which overlap the weak useful reflection. Thus, for medical diagnosis, the antenna is required to be matched to the human body. Matching the antennas on the human body (refer to human skin for the on-body matched antenna) has the purpose of reducing the strong reflection on the air-skin interface and to allow more energy to be radiated into the human body for obtaining a stronger signal for processing.

Though the implantable antennas and on-body matched antennas are used for different medical applications, their common ground is that they are both matched to the human body and are termed as **body-matched antennas** in this thesis. Therefore, the body-matched antennas refer to both the implantable and on-body matched antennas. Many challenges arise for the body-matched antennas in terms of the design, characterization, fabrication and verification, which are briefly discussed in the following paragraphs.

The design of body-matched antennas differs from that for the regular antennas for free-space operation. This is because it suffers from the problems of lossy human tissues and their different permittivities resulting in totally different wave propagation behavior. The geometry and dielectric properties of the human body must be considered for the optimization and characterization of these antennas. Therefore, the performance of the antennas (e.g. impedance matching, bandwidth, radiation pattern, etc.) is strongly dependent on the dielectric properties of tissues and structure of the human body. As a result, the antennas will suffer from reduced efficiency, radiation pattern fragmentation and variations in feed-point impedance.

Since the antennas are placed directly on or in the human body, the radiation into a multilayer lossy medium must be considered. The computational load of the simulation of the antenna model together with the human body becomes very large in terms of computer memory. The design procedure then becomes more complicated than in the case of simple free-space operation scenarios. Moreover, the size of the antennas strongly affects the performance of diagnosis imaging systems or the size of IMDs. Thus miniaturization techniques are required to significantly reduce the size of the radiating structures. Furthermore, many features such as having low profile (fabrication complexity), low weight and low cost are required for medical applications.

The characterization of the body-matched antennas must be done with the consideration of the dielectric properties of human tissues. Thus, the antenna cannot be verified in an anechoic chamber. The verification in the measurement taking into account the presence of the human body (e.g. using tissue-simulating liquid) becomes also sophisticated and the results change with the scenarios and setups. Regarding the radiation regulation for the human body, many requirements (i.e. Specific Absorption Rate (SAR) value) must also be fulfilled.

1.3. Goal and organization of this work

The goal of this work is to design body-matched antennas for the microwave healthcare system for nursing home residents (see in Figure 1.2). The focus is to miniaturize the antenna size yet maintaining high efficiency, high gain as well as stable radiation pattern over the frequency of the implantable and on-body matched antennas. The operational frequencies of the antennas range from 0.5 GHz to 10 GHz and the different frequency bands corresponding to the different applications will be given in the following chapters. With regard to the design of antennas, planar antennas are chosen due to an easy fabrication and to achieve low profile as well as low-cost devices. The miniaturization techniques of the antenna design in this thesis relies on the optimization of the feeding- and antenna structures as well as regulation of the current distribution on the radiating elements. With these achievements, it is expected that these antennas will significantly enhance the performance of the IMDs as well as imaging systems for diagnosis and thus contribute very positively to the future microwave telemedicine systems.

With this goal in mind, the organization of this work is outlined (referring to Figure 1.2) as follows:

Before the design of the body-matched antennas is introduced, the dielectric properties of the different human tissues and human model are studied in chapter 2. Based on the dielectric properties of human tissues, the microwave propagation in the human body is then investigated with respect to their reflection, attenuation and transmission. A model of the human bladder with different tissue layers including frequency dependent dielectric properties is applied for the estimation of the required SNR and dynamic range of the imaging system. In the following chapter, different characterization methods of the body-matched antennas are described. For the verification of the body-matched antennas, two antenna measurement systems with tissue-simulating liquid are given, which allow the measurements of the near-field and far-field radiation pattern of the body-matched antennas. Chapter 4 provides the design and the miniaturization concepts of implantable antennas for IMDs. That is followed by on-body matched antennas for microwave imaging at different operational frequency bands in chapter 5. The main focus is the miniaturization of the antennas without the significant degradation of the antenna performance. The applicability of the on-body matched antennas for microwave imaging is shown in Chapter 6, by means of a measurement demonstrator for the detection of the hemorrhagic stroke. Finally, Chapter 7 gives conclusions of this thesis to microwave medical applications.

2. Analysis of microwave propagation in a multilayer human body

In the modeling of the human body for microwave medical applications, the human body must be considered as a multilayer model consisting of different lossy human tissues. The human tissues are in general frequency dispersive, meaning that they distort the signal when it propagates through them. Therefore, it is of great importance to analyze the microwave propagation in the human body taking into account the frequency dependent dielectric properties of different tissues.

This chapter provides the investigation of the propagation characteristics of the electromagnetic (EM) signals in tissues. For that purpose, the dielectric properties of different tissues are analyzed. A full consideration of the propagation characteristics of the signals (from 1 to 10 GHz) in human tissues with respect to the frequency dispersion, attenuation, reflection and transmission is provided. Then, with the above knowledge, the performance as well as challenges for the microwave medical system are analyzed with a realistic human abdomen model for the detection of urine accumulation. Regarding the frequency band used, the ultra wideband (UWB) pulse from 3.1 to 10.6 GHz according to [FCC02] is investigated in terms of attenuation and distortion. Based on these results, the optimal operational frequency bands are discussed for different medical applications. This chapter ends with a short conclusion about microwave propagation in the human body and the requirements of antenna characteristics for the optimal system performance for microwave medical applications.

2.1. Microwave propagation in a lossy medium

In general, a homogeneous, isotropic and lossy medium can be described with a complex permittivity $\underline{\varepsilon}$ and permeability $\underline{\mu}$, which can be written as

$$\underline{\varepsilon} = \varepsilon' - j\varepsilon'', \tag{2.1}$$

$$\underline{\mu} = \mu' - j\mu'', \tag{2.2}$$

where ε'' and μ'' describe the dielectric loss and magnetization loss, respectively. μ'' is not considered in this thesis (assumed to be 0), since it does not exist in biological tissues. Furthermore, assuming that the human tissues are non-magnetic [VRK06], the permeability can be written as $\underline{\mu} = \mu_0$.

With regard to the permittivity, there are the loss due to dielectric damping of vibrating dipole moments and the conductive loss (or Joule loss) [Poz, ZL07]. However, it is impossible to distinguish between these losses. Since the conduction current is dominant in most biological tissues, the dielectric damping is assumed to be 0 and hence the loss is specified only by the effective conductivity loss.

Assuming that the medium has a conductivity σ, a conduction current density $\vec{J}$ exists and together with dielectric flux density $\vec{D}$, can be written as

$$\vec{J} = \sigma\vec{E}, \tag{2.3}$$

$$\vec{D} = \varepsilon_0\varepsilon_\mathrm{r}\vec{E}, \tag{2.4}$$

where E is the electric field intensity, ε_0 and ε_r is the permittivity of free space and the relative permittivity of a lossy medium, respectively. Taking into account the time varying nature of the electromagnetic waves, the electric field (E-field) intensity is described as

$$\vec{E}(x,y,z,t) = \vec{E}(x,y,z)\,e^{j\omega t}, \tag{2.5}$$

where $\omega = 2\pi f$ is the angular frequency and f is the frequency.

Based on (2.3) and (2.4), the Maxwell's equation in differential form for magnetic field intensity $\vec{H}$ can be modified to

$$
\begin{aligned}
\nabla \times \vec{H} &= \frac{\partial \vec{D}}{\partial t} + \vec{J} \\
&= j\omega\varepsilon_0\varepsilon_\mathrm{r}\vec{E} + \sigma\vec{E} \\
&= j\omega\varepsilon_0 \left[\varepsilon_\mathrm{r} - j\frac{\sigma}{\omega\varepsilon_0} \right] \vec{E}.
\end{aligned}
\tag{2.6}
$$

Thus, the complex permittivity can be modified as

$$
\underline{\varepsilon} = \varepsilon_0 \left(\varepsilon_\mathrm{r} - j\frac{\sigma}{\omega\varepsilon_0} \right).
\tag{2.7}
$$

The loss tangent can be calculated by

$$
\tan\delta = \frac{\sigma}{\omega\varepsilon_\mathrm{r}\varepsilon_0}.
\tag{2.8}
$$

Consider now the Maxwell's differential form equation for $\vec{E}$

$$
\nabla \times \vec{E} = -\frac{\partial \vec{B}}{\partial t} = -j\omega\mu_0\vec{H},
\tag{2.9}
$$

assuming that the medium is source-free, the wave equation for $\vec{E}$ can be obtained by modifying (2.9) as follows:

$$
\begin{aligned}
\nabla \times \nabla \times \vec{E} &= \nabla \times \left(-j\omega\mu_0\vec{H} \right) = -j\omega\mu_0\nabla \times \vec{H} \\
\nabla\left(\nabla\cdot\vec{E}\right) - \nabla^2\vec{E} &= \omega^2\mu_0\varepsilon_0 \left[\varepsilon_\mathrm{r} - j\frac{\sigma}{\omega\varepsilon_0} \right] \vec{E} \\
\nabla^2\vec{E} + \omega^2\mu_0\varepsilon_0 \left[\varepsilon_\mathrm{r} - j\frac{\sigma}{\omega\varepsilon_0} \right] \vec{E} &= 0.
\end{aligned}
\tag{2.10}
$$

To simplify (2.10), the wave number in lossy medium can be written as

$$
k = \omega\sqrt{\mu_0\varepsilon_0 \left[\varepsilon_\mathrm{r} - j\frac{\sigma}{\omega\varepsilon_0} \right]}.
\tag{2.11}
$$

Having the wave number k, the complex propagation constant for the medium can be then determined by

$$\gamma = \alpha + j\beta = jk = j\omega \sqrt{\mu_0 \varepsilon_0 \left[\varepsilon_r - j \frac{\sigma}{\omega \varepsilon_0} \right]}, \qquad (2.12)$$

where α and β are respectively the attenuation constant and phase constant. Separating the real and the imaginary part of the complex propagation constant yields two terms:

$$\alpha = \frac{\omega}{c_0} \sqrt{\frac{\varepsilon_r}{2} \left[\sqrt{1 + \left(\frac{\sigma}{\omega \varepsilon_0 \varepsilon_r} \right)^2} - 1 \right]}, \qquad (2.13)$$

$$\beta = \frac{\omega}{c_0} \sqrt{\frac{\varepsilon_r}{2} \left[\sqrt{1 + \left(\frac{\sigma}{\omega \varepsilon_0 \varepsilon_r} \right)^2} + 1 \right]}. \qquad (2.14)$$

It can be seen that the conductive loss results in a non-zero attenuation constant and also modifies the phase constant.

After introducing the attenuation constant α and phase constant β, the following terms will be discussed with regard to a lossy medium.

Wavelength

The wavelength of a propagating signal in a lossy medium can be written as

$$\lambda_m = \frac{2\pi}{\beta} = 2\pi c_0 / \left(\omega \sqrt{\frac{\varepsilon_r}{2} \left[\sqrt{1 + \left(\frac{\sigma}{\omega \varepsilon_0 \varepsilon_r} \right)^2} + 1 \right]} \right). \qquad (2.15)$$

Penetration depth

The penetration depth δ_p describes the penetration ability of EM waves into a lossy medium. This is defined as the depth, at the point where the amplitude of the field decreased to $1/e$ of the original value and can be described by

$$\delta_{\mathrm{p}} = \frac{1}{\alpha} = \frac{c_0}{\omega \sqrt{\frac{\varepsilon_{\mathrm{r}}}{2}\left[\sqrt{1+\left(\frac{\sigma}{\omega\varepsilon_0\varepsilon_{\mathrm{r}}}\right)^2}-1\right]}}. \tag{2.16}$$

Attenuation

Assuming that the waves propagate in the +z direction, the attenuation of the E-field (in the z direction) can be written as

$$D_{\mathrm{a}} = \frac{|E(z)|}{|E(0)|} = \frac{|E(0)| \cdot e^{-\alpha z}}{|E(0)|} = e^{-\alpha z}, \tag{2.17}$$

where the attenuation in dB is:

$$D_{\mathrm{a}}|_{\mathrm{dB}} = 20 \cdot \log_{10}\left(e^{-\alpha z}\right) = z \cdot \alpha \cdot 20 \cdot \log_{10}(e) = 8.686 \cdot \alpha \cdot z. \tag{2.18}$$

Therefore the attenuation constant in dB is expressed as $8.686 \cdot \alpha$.

Wave impedance

The wave impedance in a lossy medium is also modified to reflect a complex value:

$$Z_{\mathrm{m}} = \sqrt{\frac{\mu}{\varepsilon}} = \sqrt{\frac{\mu_0}{\varepsilon_0\left[\varepsilon_{\mathrm{r}} - j\frac{\sigma}{\omega\varepsilon_0}\right]}}. \tag{2.19}$$

Since wideband signals are in the scope of this thesis, the frequency dispersion cannot be neglected. The complex permittivity of a lossy medium from (2.7) can thus be modified to

$$\underline{\varepsilon}(\omega) = \varepsilon_0\left[\varepsilon_{\mathrm{r}}(\omega) - j\frac{\sigma(\omega)}{\omega\varepsilon_0}\right], \tag{2.20}$$

where the $\varepsilon_{\mathrm{r}}(\omega)$ and $\sigma(\omega)$ are the frequency dependent relative permittivity and conductivity, respectively.

In conclusion, the attenuation constant α, the phase constant β and the wave impedance can be determined if the complex permittivity (dielectric property) is known. Since the complex permittivities of different human tissues are the basis for the analysis of the microwave propagation in the human body, they will be introduced in the following sections.

2.2. Dielectric properties of human tissues

The dielectric properties of human tissues describe the level of interaction of the EM waves with the molecules of the tissues. For the numerical analysis of the propagation of EM waves in tissues or for determining the specific absorption rates (SAR) i.e. the absorption of EM energy by the tissues, the dielectric properties of human tissues are the key parameters. Therefore, it is of significance to determine the dielectric properties of human tissues. For that purpose, the well-known Debye equation and the Cole-Cole equation [GGC96, GLG96b], which predict the permittivity of human tissues based on experimental data of human tissues, will be introduced in the following section.

2.2.1. Debye equation and Cole-Cole equation

The dielectric properties of human tissues are frequency dependent due to the frequency-dependent (dispersion) polarization of atoms, electrons and ions caused by the E-fields in tissues [Rei98, MD99].
Assuming that an ideal, noninteracting dipoles are considered in a dielectric relaxation respons, the frequency dispersion of the dielectric properties of human tissues can be described by the well-known Debye equation [Deb60]:

$$\underline{\varepsilon} = \varepsilon_0 \left(\varepsilon_r - j \frac{\sigma}{\omega \varepsilon_0} \right) = \varepsilon_\infty + \frac{\varepsilon_s - \varepsilon_\infty}{1 + j\omega\tau'}, \tag{2.21}$$

where ε_∞ and ε_s are the permittivity at $\omega \to \infty$ (highest frequency) and $\omega \to 0$ (lowest frequency), respectively. τ' is the relaxation time, which is the required time for a stimulated dipole to return to its original state. It must be emphasized that only a single relaxation time (first order approximation of different relaxation regions, which will be mentioned in the next paragraph) is considered in this equation. Thus, the Debye equation is not sufficient to predict the dispersion in a wide frequency range. In reality, several types of relaxation processes with regard to different polarizations exist. The relaxation process can hence be extended to a wider frequency range.

The dielectric behavior of human tissue in a broadband frequency range can be separated into four dispersion regions (three main relaxation regions: dispersion for low, medium and high frequencies respectively; one minor region) classified according to the different mechanisms of polarization [Hur85]. Based on many reported experimental data of various tissues, the Cole-Cole equation [GGC96] [GLG96a] [GLG96b], which is the improved version of the Debye equation, provides multiple dispersion terms. These terms predict the frequency dependency within each dispersion region.

The Cole-Cole equation is given in (2.22), where α_n is the distribution parameter (a measure of the broadening of the dispersion) and n indicates four different dispersion regions, $\Delta\varepsilon = \varepsilon_s - \varepsilon_\infty$ denotes the magnitude of the dispersion, σ_i is the static ionic conductivity.

$$\underline{\varepsilon}(\omega) = \varepsilon_0 \left(\varepsilon_r - j\frac{\sigma}{\omega\varepsilon_0} \right) = \varepsilon_\infty + \sum_n \frac{\Delta\varepsilon_n}{1 + \left(j\omega\tau_n'\right)^{(1-\alpha_n)}} + \frac{\sigma_i}{j\omega\varepsilon_0}. \quad (2.22)$$

2.2.2. Permittivity of human tissues

Based on the Cole-Cole equation, the permittivity of different tissues can be predicted in a wideband frequency range (relevant frequency range in this thesis is from 1 to 10 GHz) (Parameters referring to appendix A). Since the detection of urine accumulation in the human bladder and the detection of stroke are within the scope of this thesis, the dielectric properties of eight types of tissues (muscle, skin, bone, fat, skull, white matter, grey matter and blood) are generated from the Cole-Cole equation. The dielectric properties of human urine and distilled water on the other hand, were measured with the Agilent 85070E Dielectric Probe Kit.

Figure 2.1 (a) shows the relative permittivity (ε_r) of these ten tissues over frequency. Starting with the tissues which have the lowest relative permittivity, fat has the lowest relative permittivity of around 5, since its water content is almost negligible. Furthermore, the dispersion of the permittivity of fat is not remarkable in the frequency range from 1 to 10 GHz. This is followed by the skull (cortical bone) and bone. At 5 GHz, the skull has a relative permittivity of 10, while that of the bone is around 18.

The ε_r of white matter, skin, grey matter and muscle are between 30 and 50. They have a large relative permittivity due to the high water content present in these tissues. Grey matter exhibits a slightly higher relative permittivity than white matter. Those with the relative permittivity of above 50 are blood, urine and distilled water. Water and urine show similar relative permittivity between 70 and 80. It can also be seen that the frequency dependency of the relative permittivity of tissues with high water content varies very significantly over the 1 to 10 GHz range.

From Figure 2.1 (a), it can be concluded that the blood in the human brain and the urine in human bladder have high relative permittivity compared to their surrounding tissues. This high contrast of relative permittivity to the surrounding tissues provides the potential for detecting the position or volume of the blood and urine accumulation in the human body.

The losses of the respective materials are related to the conductivity as shown in Figure 2.1 (b). Fat, skull, bone and white matter exhibit a low conductivity, while the respective quantities for water, urine, blood and muscle show larger values. Urine and blood have high conductivities of 7.5 and 5.5 S/m at 5 GHz, respectively. Therefore, a large attenuation of the EM signals in water, urine and muscle is expected. The conductivity of urine is higher than that of distilled water. This is because urine contains more ions and electrons than distilled water and this results in a higher conductivity. Furthermore, it must be noted that the frequency dependency on the conductivity of the tissues with high water content is very strong from 1 to 10 GHz. This is because the vibrating distance of ions becomes shorter with increasing frequency and hence the conductivity is improved.

2.2.3. Attenuation, penetration depth and wave impedance in human tissues

Based on the complex relative permittivity of different human tissues, the attenuation constant and penetration depth of EM waves in these tissues can be determined using (2.13) and (2.16) to investigate the influence of the conduc-

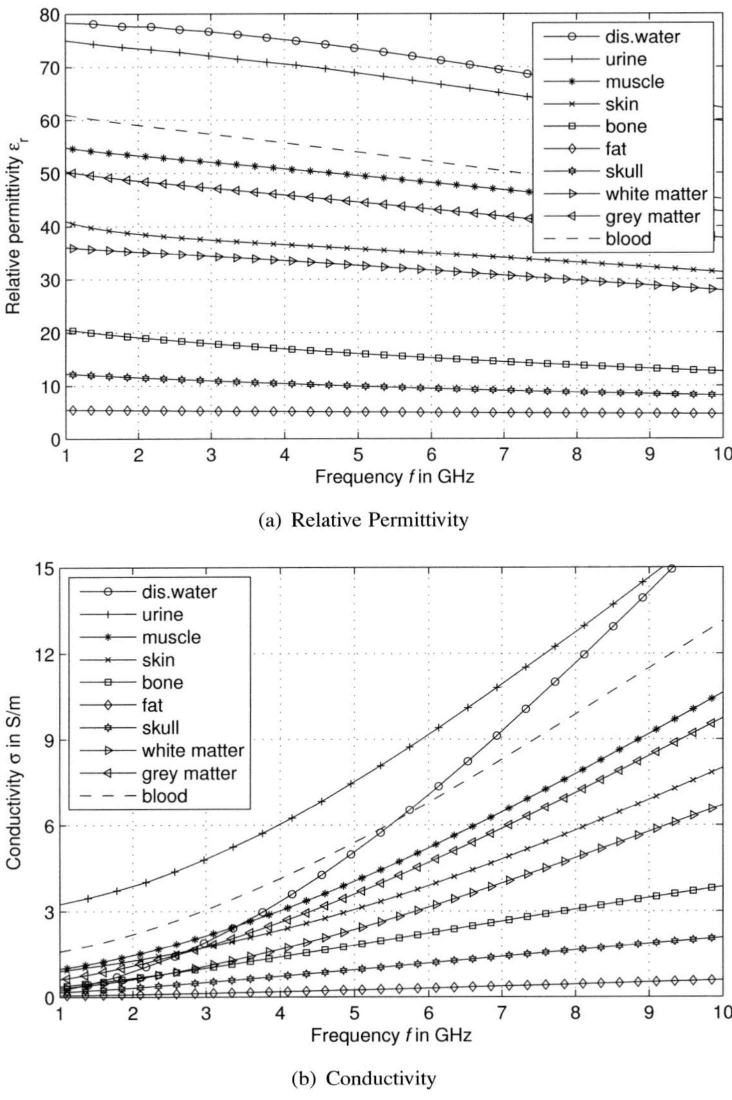

(a) Relative Permittivity

(b) Conductivity

Figure 2.1.: Relative permittivity and conductivity of different human tissues over frequency (distilled water and urine: measured by the author; other tissues: predicted by the Cole-Cole equation).

tivity on the microwave propagation. In Figure 2.2, the attenuation constant and penetration depth related to different tissues are presented.

The results show that EM waves typically undergo much higher attenuation in human tissues than in free space, e.g. attenuation constant caused by oxygen absorption and water vapor absorption at 1 GHz being 8×10^{-8} and 1×10^{-8} dB/cm [LHC93], respectively. However, the attenuation constant caused by fat, bone and white matter at 1 GHz is around 1 dB/cm. The tissues with high water content (muscle, blood and urine) show a higher attenuation constant. Furthermore, this value increases strongly with frequency, which introduces distortion for wideband signals due to the different signal attenuations at different frequencies. This is investigated quantitatively in section 2.3 with respect to the fidelity of an ultra wideband (UWB) pulse.

The high signal attenuation caused by human tissues reduces the performance of any kind of microwave system for medical applications, where signal penetration into and reflection from the tissues are required. Figure 2.2 (b) shows that the signal from 1 to 3 GHz has a large penetration depth in different tissues (e.g. 4 cm in muscle at 1 GHz), while at above 5 GHz δ_p decreases (1 cm in muscle at 5 GHz). Therefore, a very high system dynamic range is required to capture the weak reflections from the tissues at high frequencies. Moreover, the different attenuations of the signal at different frequencies result in the distortion of the frequency spectrum of the received signal. The received signal level can be very different over a wider frequency range (e.g. the whole UWB frequency range from 3.1 to 10.6 GHz according to [FCC02]), which must be considered in the design of the system.

After the discussion about the attenuation and penetration depth of microwave signal in different human tissues, the wave impedance in tissues is analyzed. This is of significance for the impedance matching of the body-matched antennas in the later chapters. Taking a plane wave for example, the wave impedance of a plane wave in different human tissues becomes complex due to the complex permittivity of the tissues. For the purpose of comparison, only the absolute value of the wave impedance is provided in Figure 2.3. The values in all tissues are much lower than in free space (Z_{F0}=377 Ω). In this case, the impedance matching from the 50 Ω feed line of the antennas to a low wave impedance in tissues can be easily achieved. However, the different

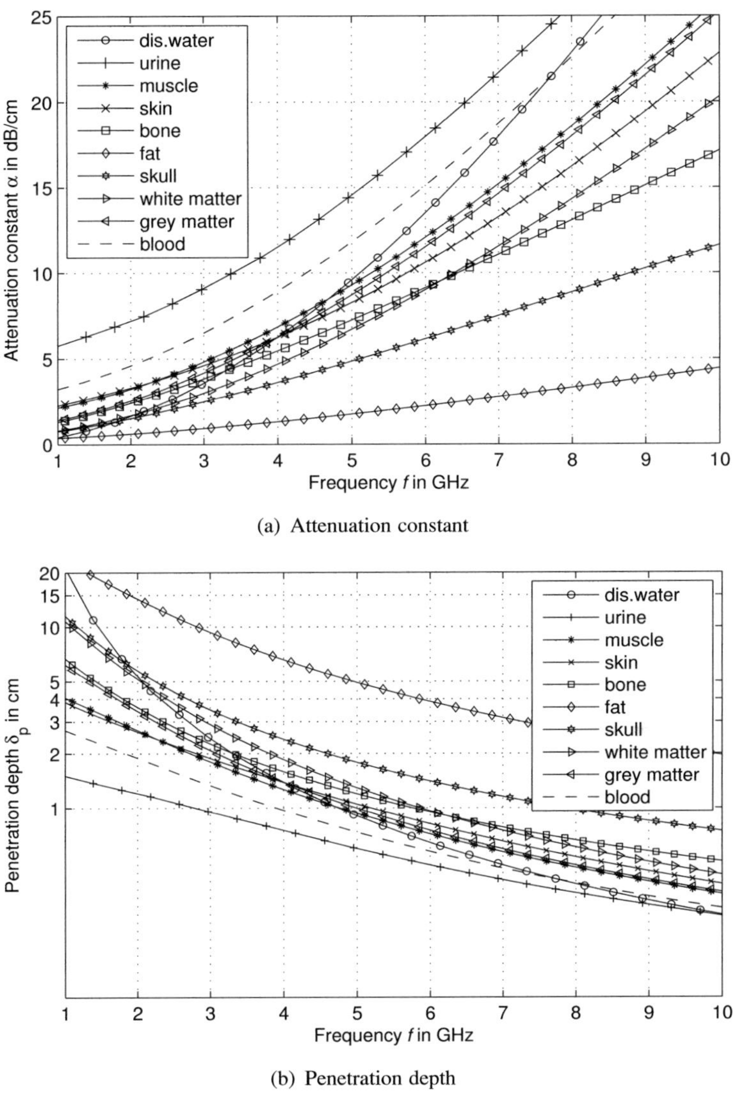

(a) Attenuation constant

(b) Penetration depth

Figure 2.2.: Attenuation constant and penetration depth of microwaves in different human tissues over frequency.

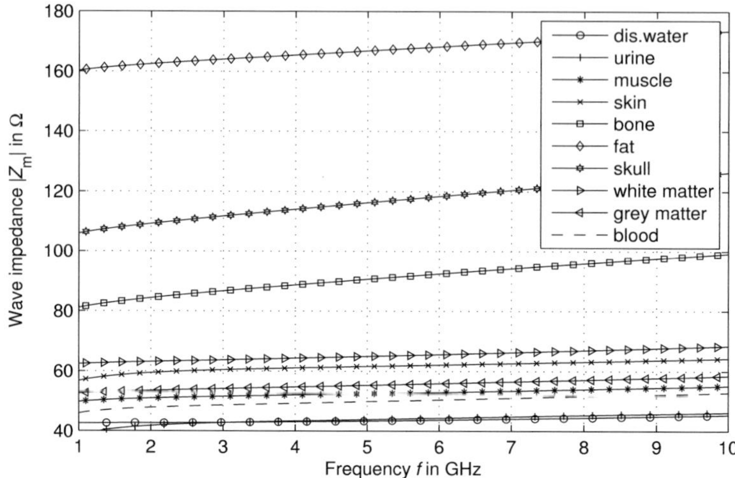

Figure 2.3.: Wave impedance in different human tissues over frequency.

wave impedances in different tissues result in different impedance matchings for a given body-matched antenna. Therefore, the impedance matching of the antennas placed in different tissues will be changed strongly. The resulted impedance mismatch reduced considerably the radiation efficiency of the body-matched antennas.

With the knowledge of the dielectric properties of different human tissues as well as the corresponding quantities (such as attenuation, penetration depth and wave impedance), the microwave propagation in the human body consisting of different tissues can now be analyzed.

2.3. Analysis of microwave propagation in the human bladder

In this section, urine detection in the human bladder motivates the analysis of the propagation of microwave signals (GHz range) in the human body. The detection and the monitoring of urine in the human bladder is of significance in medical fields and has been discussed in the introduction. It can be achieved by detecting the reflected microwave signals from the boundaries of human tissues such as fat and bladder muscle. Thus, the microwave signals have to penetrate different tissues of the abdomen. Due to the high attenuation and frequency dispersion of the microwave signals in human tissues, the detection possibility of the reflected signals is strongly degraded. Therefore, a quantitative investigation of the microwave propagation in the human body is significant for the prediction of performance of microwave medical systems also to help design more effective antenna systems to counter the propagation loss.

Based on the dielectric properties of the different human tissues introduced in the last section, the propagation characteristics of microwave signals are investigated with respect to their reflection, attenuation and transmission. A model of the human bladder with different tissue layers including the frequency dependent dielectric properties is used. Furthermore, a system concept of the UWB radar for the detection of water accumulation in the human bladder is introduced. The UWB pulse attenuation and distortion in different human tissues are then investigated and evaluated.

2.3.1. Multilayer model of the human abdomen

Since the permittivity of different human tissues has been investigated, a multilayer model of the human abdomen with realistic dielectric properties can be implemented. According to the Visible Human Project male dataset [USNLoM], a multilayer structure of the human abdomen can be modeled as shown in Figure 2.4. This dielectric model consists of 6 different layers of human tissues. The connective tissue between skin and muscle is modeled as fat, since it is composed mostly of fatty tissue. To simplify this model for the analysis excluding a sophisticated geometry, each layer is assumed to be flat. The typical thickness of each tissue is based on the investigations on adults (20-60 years old) [CKK04] and are summarized in Table 2.1.

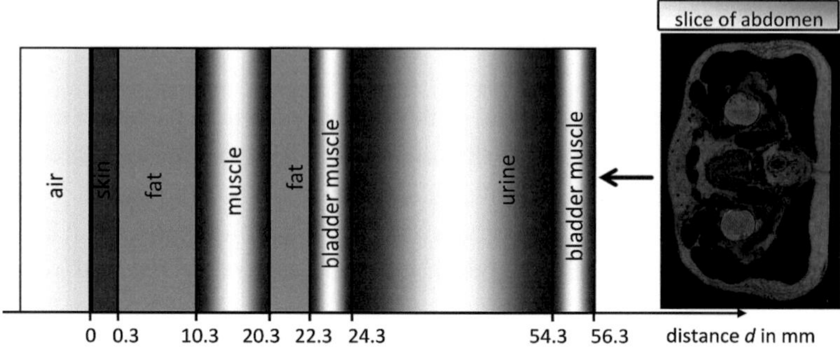

Figure 2.4.: Multilayer model of human abdomen.

Table 2.1.: Typical thicknesses of tissues in the human abdomen (full bladder) based on adults between 20-60 years old.

tissue	thickness (mm)
skin	0.3
connective tissue (fat)	10
muscle	10
fat	2
bladder muscle	2
urine	30
bladder muscle	2

2.3.2. Concept of the radar system

For the analysis of microave propagation in the human bladder, an appropriate concept of radar system is required. In [1], [22, 23], the system performance of three different radar concepts with different signal modulations were investigated by the author. They are impulse-radio (IR) approach, frequency sweep approach with Vector Network Analyzer (VNA) (details will be given in chapter 6) and the Pseudo-noise (PN) approach. These concepts are widely used under the research for medical applications in the recent years. The performance of these three radar concepts have been verified in measurements by the author. It has been found that the impulse-radio (IR) approach has the lowest system dynamic range of the three radar systems, but it also has the lowest system complexity [Vat10]. Using the frequency sweep approach with VNA and the Pseudo-noise (PN) approach a high system dynamic range can be achieved [Sch10].

To obtain the characteristics of microwave propagation in the human abdomen, the analysis both in the time and the frequency domain (for the IR approach and the frequency sweep approach, respectively) is considered in the following section.

With regard to the IR approach, the UWB pulse with a frequency range from 3.1 to 10.6 GHz is used. The block diagram of the proposed Impulse-Radio Ultra Wideband (IR-UWB) radar system is shown in Figure 2.5. The transmitter consists of a trigger, a pulse generator and a transmit antenna. The signal is received by a separate antenna, which is connected to a sampling unit. The reflected signal is sampled by a device with a high sampling rate and a data acquisition unit. In this IR-UWB concept, a correlation analysis in the time domain is performed to enhance the SNR of the received signal. For that purpose, the received UWB signal is correlated with the reference signal from the transmitter. Since the human tissues are dispersive materials, the received signal is distorted as it propagates through the tissues, which results in a degraded correlation function between transmitted and received pulses. The degradation of the received UWB pulse can be evaluated in terms of distortion and fidelity. The distortion d_p is mathematically defined as the variation of the received signal $u_R(t)$ with respect to the transmitted signal $u_T(t)$ [LS94]:

$$d_\mathrm{p} = \min_\tau \int_{-\infty}^{+\infty} \left| \frac{u_R(t+\tau)}{\left[\int_{-\infty}^{+\infty} |u_R(t)|^2 \right]^{1/2}} - \frac{u_T(t)}{\left[\int_{-\infty}^{+\infty} |u_T(t)|^2 \right]^{1/2}} \right|^2 dt. \quad (2.23)$$

Based on the distortion, F_p quantifies the fidelity of the received pulse compared to the transmitted signal and is determined by the peak of the cross-correlation function as

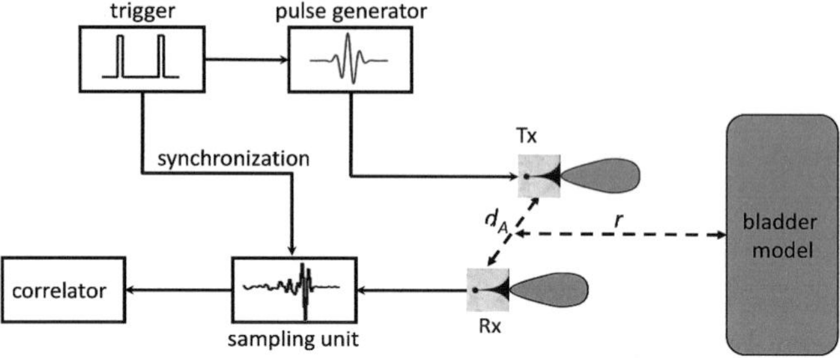

Figure 2.5.: Block diagram of the IR-UWB radar system for urine detection in the human bladder (d_A: distance between transmitting and receiving antennas; r: distance between antennas and bladder model).

$$F_p = \max_\tau \int_{-\infty}^{+\infty} \frac{u_R(t + \tau)}{\left[\int_{-\infty}^{+\infty} |u_R(t)|^2\right]^{1/2}} \cdot \frac{u_T(t)}{\left[\int_{-\infty}^{+\infty} |u_T(t)|^2\right]^{1/2}} dt. \qquad (2.24)$$

Since the sign of the correlation can be usually neglected, the absolute value of F_p is used. It can be concluded that the minimum distortion is obtained when the fidelity between the two signals is maximum.

With the introduction of the model of the human abdomen and the related radar concepts, the characteristics of microwave propagation can be analyzed as shown in the following sections.

2.3.3. Characteristics of propagating microwave signals in the multilayer abdomen

During the propagation of microwave signals in the human abdomen, reflections occur at the boundaries of different tissues. The magnitude of the UWB signals is dependent on the dielectric contrast of tissues. The reflection coefficient of the plane wave can be determined using the Fresnel equation. In the case of normal incidence to the surface of the two dielectrics, whose permittivities are denoted as $\underline{\varepsilon}_1$ and $\underline{\varepsilon}_2$, the normal incident reflection coefficient can be written as

$$\Gamma = \frac{\sqrt{\varepsilon_1} - \sqrt{\varepsilon_2}}{\sqrt{\varepsilon_1} + \sqrt{\varepsilon_2}}. \tag{2.25}$$

Microwave signals propagating through the multilayer model of the human abdomen (refer to Figure 2.4) will experience reflections at the boundaries between the various tissues. The reflection (calculated by 2.25) and transmission properties of microwave signals at the boundaries of different tissues are shown in Figure 2.6. An analysis is performed in the frequency domain (from 1 to 10 GHz) for a better comparison. The first strong reflection occurs at the boundary between air and skin, where half of the energy is reflected back. Since the contrast between skin and fat as well as between fat and muscle are very high, strong reflections are also caused at these two boundaries. The reflection from the boundary between the muscle and urine is weak, since the two tissues show little difference in the dielectric property. The bladder muscle has a thickness of approximately 0.2 mm and has a low contrast with respect to urine. Hence for the detection of urine in the human bladder, the reflection from the boundary between fat and bladder muscle can be used directly.

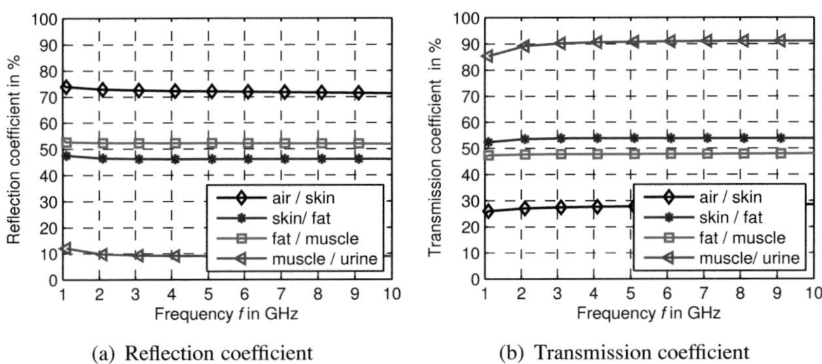

(a) Reflection coefficient   (b) Transmission coefficient

Figure 2.6.: Simulated reflection and transmission coefficient of different tissue boundaries over frequency (The frequency dependance of dielectric property is included).

The signal attenuation, the penetration depth and the attenuation constant of 4 human tissues (skin, fat, muscle and urine) in the frequency range from 1 to 10 GHz are shown in Figure 2.2. In the fat tissue the signal has a penetration depth of 9.3 cm at 3 GHz, while a penetration depth of around 1.9 cm in skin tissue is identified. In urine, an extremely low penetration depth (0.95 cm at 3 GHz) is observed. The value, as expected, decreases with increasing frequency. At 8 GHz a penetration depth of 2.6 cm in the fat tissue is noted.

In Figure 2.2 (a) the attenuation constant of different tissues is shown. It provides an estimate of the amount of the signal attenuation during propagation through the tissues. The results show that e.g. urine has an attenuation of 9.1 dB/cm at 3 GHz, which increases up to 25.6 dB/cm at 8 GHz. The signal attenuation in the skin and muscle tissue are also very high (at 4.6 dB/cm and 4.8 dB/cm at 3 GHz, respectively). The fat tissue causes relatively low signal attenuation while its attenuation constant is 0.91 dB/cm at 3 GHz. The reason for this is the low water content in fat.

2.3.4. Distortion and fidelity of UWB pulses in human tissues

In the IR-UWB system, the correlation between the received signal and template pulse is calculated to enhance the SNR of the received signal. As has been shown, the complex permittivity of human tissues changes relatively strongly over the considered frequency range. Hence the transmitted pulse is distorted due to its large bandwidth. As a consequence the pulse undergoes changes in its form, amplitude and width. This makes the pulse detection complicated and decreases the resolution of the UWB system. Therefore, the signal distortion of UWB signals is quantitatively analyzed as follows.

In order to investigate the dispersive effect only regarding the dielectric properties of human tissues, the radiation properties of the antennas are not considered. Therefore, a plane wave is used as the excitation signal (TEM mode) in the simulation shown in Figure 2.7. The analysis is performed with a tissue-phantom of a single tissue with frequency-dependent dielectric property in the commercial software Computer Simulation Technology (CST) Microwave Studio. In the simulation, a open boundary condition is applied and the reflection at the boundary is not considered. The transmitted signal (pulse) has the frequency bandwidth from 3.1 to 10.6 GHz. Different human tissues are investigated separately. The signal is fed directly to the surface of the human tissue, which has a size of $50 \times 50 \times 100\,\text{mm}^3$. Several probes, which are placed in the tissue, are used to obtain the pulses at different distances to the feed port in the tissue.

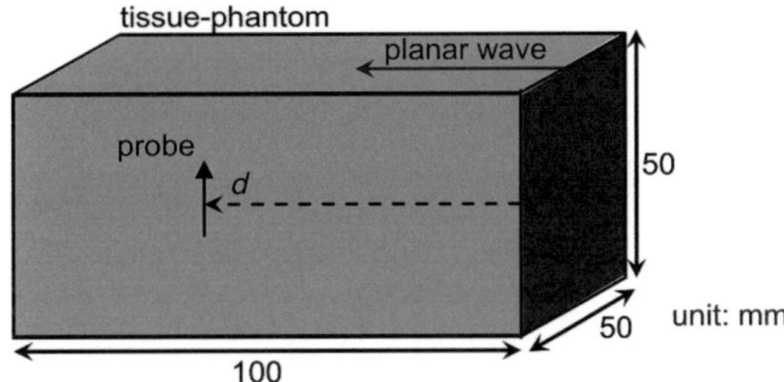

Figure 2.7.: Diagram of the simulation configuration with plane wave and probes.

Figure 2.8 (a) shows the attenuation of the transmitted pulse in human tissues. To calculate the attenuation of the pulse, the amplitude of the pulse (frequency range from 3.1 to 10.6 GHz) is evaluated. The amplitude of the pulse in the fat tissue decreases slightly as the thickness increases. A thickness of 10 mm of fat tissues causes an attenuation of 2.75 dB, while in the case of muscle and urine the resulting attenuation is 13.7 dB and 19.7 dB, respectively. It agrees with the analysis for a single frequency that the tissue with a higher water content causes higher signal attenuation. Moreover, the curves are not completely linear, since the surface waves cannot be completely eliminated in simulation. Since the presence of the surface waves must be also considered during the microwave propagation in the human body in the realistic scenario, this effect can be tolerated in this analysis.

The fidelity and distortion of the UWB pulse are shown in Figure 2.8 (b) and (c). The pulses propagating through urine, skin and muscle exhibit a strong decrease of the fidelity and an increase of the distortion with increasing thickness of the tissue. However, at a thickness of 10 mm, the fidelity of the

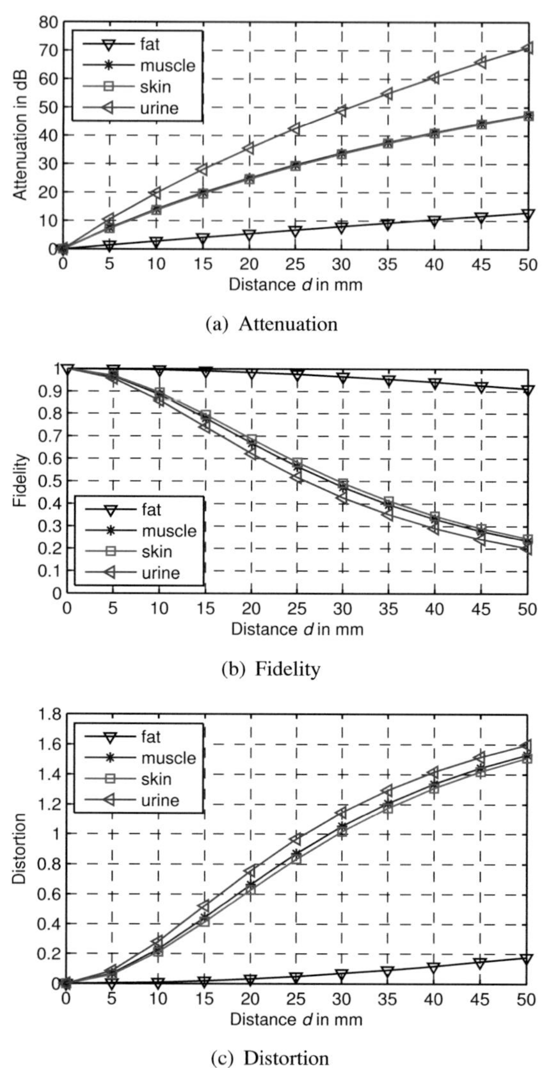

(a) Attenuation

(b) Fidelity

(c) Distortion

Figure 2.8.: Simulated attenuation, fidelity and distortion of UWB pulse in various human tissues (muscle, skin, bone, fat and distilled water).

signals in these three tissues is still better than 0.8.

In reality the tissues that cause the high distortion (i.e. skin, muscle) are relatively thin (in the range of 10 mm). The resulted fidelity is still very high (refer to Figure 2.8 (b)). On the other hand, it can be noted that the tissues with low water content (e.g. fat tissue) show very low distortion of the UWB pulse. It can therefore be concluded that although some tissues cause distortion of the signals, the effect is acceptable and the correlation receiver can be still applied for the reception of the signal.

2.3.5. Analysis of the system dynamic range for urine detection in the human bladder

After the investigation of the microwave propagation in single human tissue, the system dynamic range of the system together with the bladder model is estimated. The goal is to predict the required system dynamic range for the detection of the urine in the human bladder.

To demonstrate the frequency dependency of the radar link budget, the received signal is evaluated in the frequency domain. If the transmitted signal is denoted by $X(f)$ and the received signal by $Y(f)$, then the whole propagation process can be described with the following mathematical formula [SW05]:

$$\frac{Y(f)}{\sqrt{Z_0}} = H_{\text{Rx}}(f) \cdot H_{\text{c}}(f) \cdot H_{\text{Tx}}(f) \cdot j\omega \cdot \frac{X(f)}{\sqrt{Z_0}}, \qquad (2.26)$$

where $H_{\text{Tx}}(f)$ and $H_{\text{Rx}}(f)$ are the transfer functions of the transmitting and receiving antennas, respectively, and $H_{\text{c}}(f)$ is the channel transfer function of the scenario, which includes the propagation, reflections, dispersion and attenuation of EM waves. The reflection from each tissue boundary is taken into account. The received signal is hence a superposition of temporarily shifted echoes from all boundaries.

In the simulation model, a plane wave is used as the excitation signal. The antenna transfer functions (Tx and Rx) are then included in the model, however the near-field effect of the antennas (affecting very slightly the signal attenuation of the reflections from the boundaries of the tissues) is not considered to simplify the simulation model [Vat10], since the focus is on the estimation of the signal attenuation caused by human tissues. With this assumption the obtained transfer function of the whole system $H_s(f)$ can be written as

$$H_s(f) = \frac{Y(f)}{X(f)} = j\omega \cdot H_{\text{Tx}}(f) \cdot S \cdot \frac{e^{j\omega r/c_0}}{2\pi r c_0} \cdot H_{\text{Rx}}(f), \qquad (2.27)$$

where S is the reflection characteristic of the human abdomen model with multiple tissue layers.

It must be noted that in medical scenarios, the antennas are the critical elements of the overall system and they directly affect the recovered signals in terms of SNR and distortion. To demonstrate the best performance of the simulation model, typical Vivaldi-antennas are applied, which are matched in free space (off-body antenna). The antenna features a size of 78×75 mm^2, fed by aperture coupling and optimized for the frequency range from 2.5 to 12.5 GHz [SW05]. The transfer function of the antenna in main beam direction in the H-plane is shown in Figure 2.9. The drawbacks of the off-body antennas will be given together with the results, which will motivate the design of the on-body matched antennas in chapter 5.

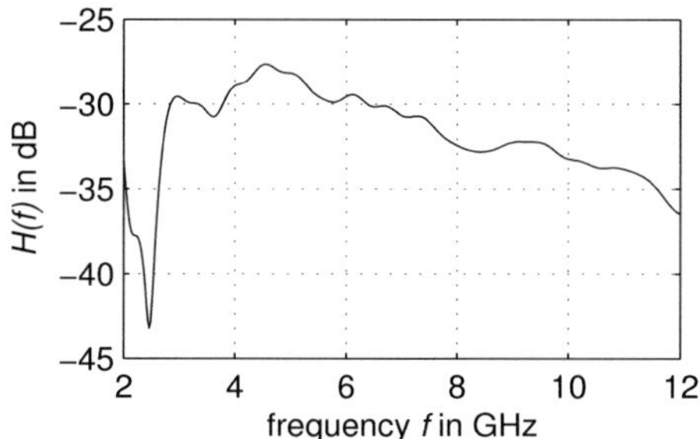

Figure 2.9.: The transfer function $H(f)$ of the used Vivaldi antenna in main beam direction, H-plane, co-polarization.

In the system concept, two identical Vivaldi antennas are used at the collocated transmitter and receiver side. The main beam of the antennas is oriented perpendicularly to the surface of the bladder model and vertical polarization is applied. The antennas are placed at a distance of 50 mm from the human abdomen model [20].

The transfer function of the whole system H_s in the considered scenario including the antenna performance, free space propagation, attenuation, reflection and transmission in human tissues at different frequencies is depicted in Figure 2.10. The initial attenuation value of lower than 0 dB results from the implementation of the term $j\omega \cdot H_{Tx}(f) \cdot \frac{e^{j\omega r/c_0}}{2\pi c_0} \cdot H_{Rx}(f)$ at the starting point ($d = $ -50 mm; antenna transfer function in the main beam direction is used). The different attenuations at the starting point at different frequencies are caused by the frequency dependency of the antenna transfer function. Furthermore, three important reflections from the boundaries between fat, bladder muscle and urine are taken into account.

At 2 GHz, the attenuation of the reflection from the boundary between fat and bladder muscle is at the level of 58 dB. The reflection from the boundary between bladder muscle and urine is estimated to 76 dB. Due to the high attenuation caused by the urine, the attenuation of the reflection from the boundary between bladder and bladder muscle (at the rear side of the bladder) is 120 dB. At 3 GHz, the reflection from the boundary between fat and bladder muscle and boundary between bladder muscle and urine are at the level of 50 dB and 70 dB, respectively. The reason for this is the higher amplitude of the antenna transfer function at 3 GHz (the antenna is optimized for the frequency range from 2.5 to 11 GHz). It must be noted that the attenuation increases strongly with increasing frequency above 3 GHz (note the scale in the case of 7 GHz). The attenuation of the reflection from the boundaries between bladder muscle and urine at 7 GHz is estimated to be 95 dB. At this level of attenuation, the reflection is difficult to be detected due to the limited sensitivity at the receiver.

The reflection from the boundaries between urine and bladder muscle (at the rear side of the bladder) in the whole frequency range is not detectable, since the attenuation is larger than 100 dB from 2 to 7 GHz. However, the reflection from the boundary between urine and bladder muscle (at the front side of the bladder) before the transmission through urine can be detected from 2 to 7 GHz. The variation of the front bladder muscle can be also utilized to estimate the volume of urine in the human bladder.

It can be also seen that a strong reflection exists at the boundary between air and skin, which introduces a reduction of 6.5 dB (incident and back-scattered

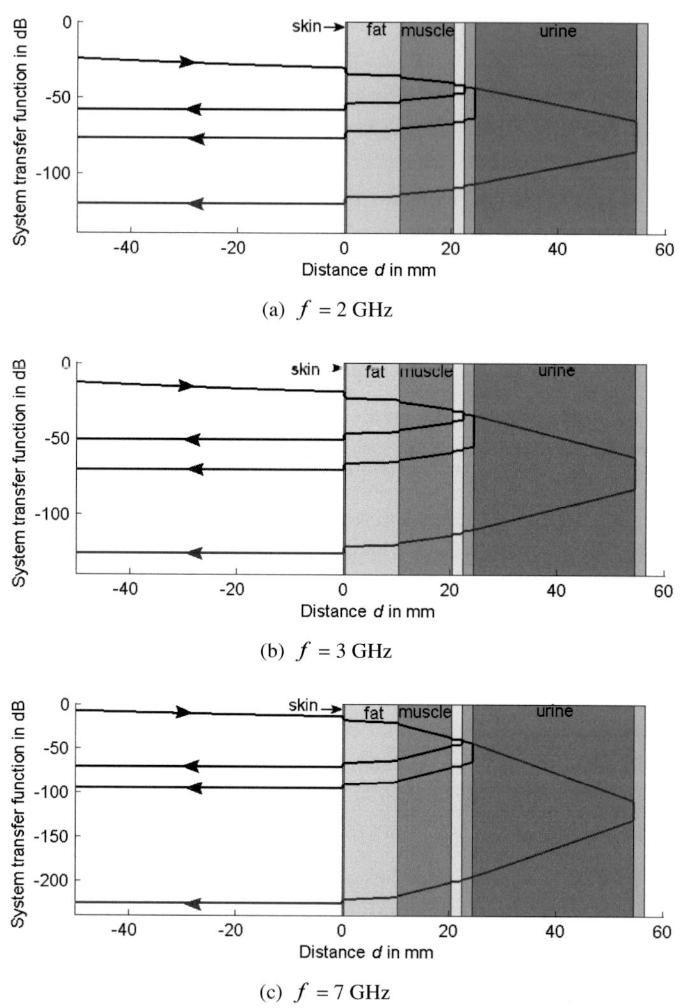

Figure 2.10.: Signal attenuation (system transfer function) of the different reflections from the boundaries in the human abdomen model (refer to Figure 2.4) at different frequencies.

wave) in the system transfer function. This indicates that 75% of the transmitted energy is scattered from the skin. The free space attenuation at a distance of 50 mm introduces a decrease of 6 dB in system transfer function. Furthermore, the problem of the mismatch of the antenna placed close to the human body has not yet been considered. Therefore, the off-body antenna causes a high decrease (> 12.5 dB) of the system transfer function.

From these results it can be concluded that a very high system dynamic range (larger than 80 dB) is needed to capture the weak reflections for the detection of urine of the human bladder, since the reflected signals after transmission through the human tissues are very weak and hardly detectable. For that purpose, the frequency sweep approach can be adopted, since a high system dynamic range can be obtained using large input power and low the noise level (using small intermediate frequency (IF) bandwidth). However, the IR approach is not suitable for this detection due to the system dynamic range being strictly limited by quantization resolution of sampling unit [Vat10].

2.4. Summary

The dielectric properties of human tissues predicted from Cole-Cole equation showed that the high water-content tissues such as muscle and urine exhibit high relative permittivity, very high signal attenuation and low penetration depth. On the other hand, the EM waves in tissues with low water-content (e.g. fat and connective tissue) undergo a low attenuation. Moreover, because of the high dielectric contrast between tissues with high and low water-content, strong reflections occur at their boundary, which can be utilized for the detection purpose.

After the quantitative study of the dielectric properties of human tissues, the performance of a microwave medical system for the detection of the urine in the human bladder, using an IR-UWB concept, has been investigated. The introduced model predicts that for a typical human body the distortion is small enough for the reception of the signal. Furthermore, the predictions of the presented model can be applied for the calibration in the radar signal processing, which further increases the performance of the system and detection capability.

In the concept for the analysis of the system dynamic range for urine detection in the human bladder, two Vivaldi-antennas matched in free space are used. The results show that there will be a decrease of at least 12.5 dB of the received signal level, using the traditional antennas matched in free space. Considering this drawback, a concept of the on-body matched antennas mentioned in the introduction arises, which can improve the microwave system performance for the medical diagnosis. More advantages of on-body matched antennas will be given in chapter 5. By using an antenna array, which will be discussed in chapter 6, the detection ability of weak reflections in such a system can be significantly improved.

With the knowledge of this feasibility study based on the model of the human abdomen for the detection of urine in the human bladder using a realistic model and parameters, the required system dynamic range and suitable frequency range can be quantitatively predicted. It has been shown in signal attenuation of reflections from the abdomen model that the UWB band from 3.1 to 10.6 GHz licensed for communication according to [FCC02] is not an optimal frequency range for microwave medical diagnosis due to the high signal attenuation in human tissues at the higher frequencies. Nevertheless, the higher frequencies are needed to enlarge the bandwidth to achieve a fine range resolution. A system dynamic range of 80 dB below 5 GHz is needed for the detection of the weak reflections at the boundary between bladder muscle and urine and is still achievable. However, the reflected signals above 7 GHz are not detectable and hence not usable. Therefore, the highest operational frequency of about 7 GHz can be considered. On the other hand, lower frequencies are preferred to be applied due to their good penetration ability. A big challenge at the lower frequencies is the large wavelength and hence large antenna size. This leads to the challenge of miniaturizing the on-body matched antennas, which will be given in chapter 5.

Regarding the suitable frequency band for on-body matched antennas in imaging systems for diagnosis, frequency bands such as 1-7 GHz or even 0.5-2 GHz for different applications are proposed (see chapter 5). For medical data transmission using microwaves, low frequencies (low signal attenuation) for implantable antennas are desirable (see chapter 4), since a long operational range is required for the wireless communication with the external devices. However, the band is constrained to be very narrow (within 100 MHz) according to the spectrum regulation of the government.

Since the body-matched antennas (on-body matched and implanted antennas) are directly in contact or embedded in the human tissues, special characterization methods and measurement systems with tissue-simulating liquid are required and will be, before the developments of different antennas, introduced in the following chapter.

3. Characterization methods and measurement systems of body-matched antennas

This chapter deals with the methods for the characterization and measurement verification of body-matched antennas. In the first section, different characterization methods of body-matched antennas are introduced to evaluate the performance of the to-be-designed antennas. Taking the lossy medium into account, the important terms of body-matched antennas are discussed.

The second part of this chapter provides the verification systems of the body-matched antennas. Since the antennas are matched to the lossy human body, the antennas have to be surrounded by a tissue-simulating liquid for the measurement verification. Due to a high signal attenuation in the tissue-simulating liquid and the increasing signal attenuation with frequency, the measurement distance and highest frequency are both limited. Therefore, two special antenna measurement systems are introduced to experimentally verify the radiation pattern of the body-matched antennas. The E-field probe based antenna measurement system allows the direct measurement of the pattern of the body-matched antennas at a short distance ($< 60\,\mathrm{mm}$). The far-field pattern of the antennas can be obtained by near-field to far-field (NF-FF) transformation of the electric near-fields, which can be measured by a planar-rectangular near-field measurement system.

3.1. Characterization methods of body-matched antennas

The analysis of antennas, which are surrounded by lossy medium is very different from the antennas in free space, since the lossy medium results in a different wavelength and introduces additional conduction current. Many quantities (e.g. wavelength, wave number, attenuation constant, phase constant, etc.) that are real in free space become complex in a lossy medium [Moo63, Kar04]. Therefore, different characterization methods of body-matched antenna such as reflection coefficient, bandwidth, efficiency and radiation pattern are provided in the following section, some of those definitions are modified for antennas in lossy medium.

3.1.1. Antenna terms in a lossy medium

Impedance and reflection coefficient

An equivalent circuit of a transmitting antenna is shown in Figure 3.1, where the antenna is fed by a feed line with characteristic impedance of Z_0. The antenna impedance can be expressed as

$$\underline{Z}_A = R_L + R_{rad} + jX_A, \qquad (3.1)$$

where R_L and R_{rad} are the loss resistance and the radiation resistance of the antenna, respectively. X_A is the reactance of antenna.

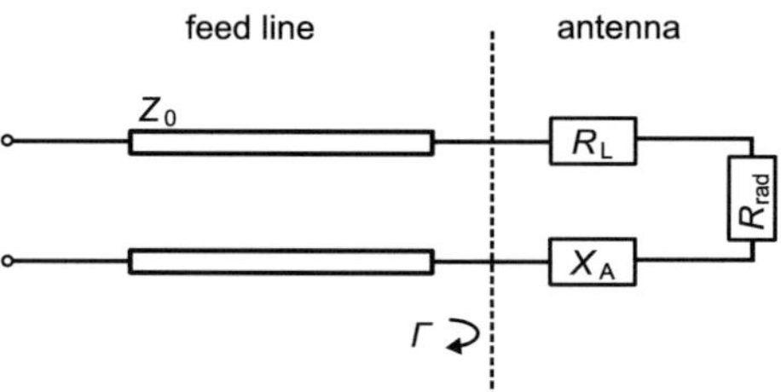

Figure 3.1.: Equivalent circuit of the transmitting antenna.

The antenna is assumed to be placed in a lossy medium with an infinitely large dimension according to the spherical coordinates shown in Figure 3.2. According to the definition in the case of the antenna in free space, the radiation resistance can be modified in terms of radiated power P_{rad} in far-field and the input current I [Bal05]:

$$R_{rad} = \frac{P_{rad}}{I^2} = \frac{\int\int S_L sin\theta\, r^2 d\theta d\varphi}{I^2},$$ (3.2)

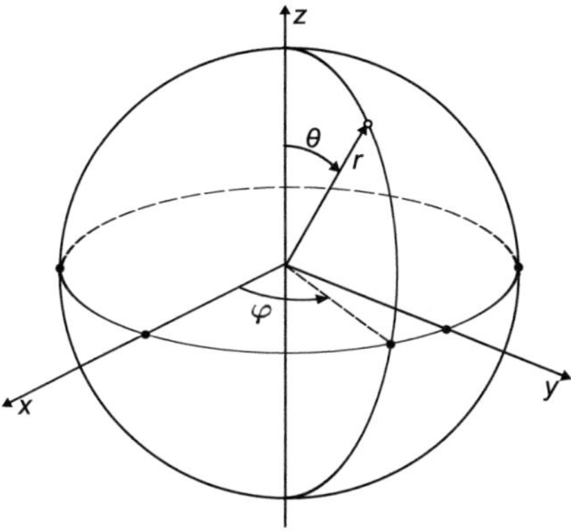

Figure 3.2.: Illustration of the spherical coordinate system.

where the power density in lossy medium S_L can be written as

$$S_L = Re\left[\frac{\left|\vec{E}\right|^2}{Z_m}\right] \cdot e^{-2\alpha r},$$ (3.3)

which is modified by introducing a decay factor $e^{2\alpha r}$ (α in lossy medium is a negative value) to compensate for the attenuation caused by the lossy medium (Z_m is the wave impedance in a lossy medium). Although the attenuation of the waves in a lossy medium is already compensated, the radiation resistance and E-field are still different compared to the one of the antenna in free space. It is because the current distribution of the antenna is altered due to the presence of the lossy medium with high relative permittivity.

With the radiation resistance and reactance of the body-matched antenna, the antenna efficiency and the reflection coefficient Γ can be determined as

$$\eta = \frac{R_{\text{rad}}}{R_{\text{rad}} + R_{\text{L}}},$$ (3.4)

$$\Gamma = \frac{\underline{Z}_{\text{A}} - Z_0}{\underline{Z}_{\text{A}} + Z_0}.$$ (3.5)

To achieve a low reflection coefficient, it is required to match the impedance of the power source with that of the antenna. Ideally, the line impedance Z_0 must be complex conjugate to the antenna's impedance $\underline{Z}_{\text{A}}$. To achieve that, in practice, various techniques e.g. matching networks are used.

The value of the magnitude of Γ is equal to the input reflection coefficient S_{11}. A good impedance matching is evaluated and compared to -10 dB regarding reflection coefficient.

Radiation pattern in near-field and far-field

The antenna radiation pattern is the specification of the angular dependence of the radiated EM waves from the antenna. Based on the spherical coordinate system (see Figure 3.2), the antenna pattern is related to the solid angles θ as well as φ and is defined with regard to the E-fields as

$$C(r,\theta,\varphi) = \left. \frac{\left|\vec{E}(r,\theta,\varphi)\right|}{\left|\vec{E}(r,\theta,\varphi)\right|_{\text{max}}} \right|_{r=\text{const.}}$$ (3.6)

Depending on the distance to the antenna, a distinction must be made between near-field and far-field radiation pattern. For that purpose, the electromagnetic field radiated by an antenna can be simplified into three characteristic regions: reactive near-field, radiating near-field and far-field.

The reactive near-field (Rayleigh zone) is caused by charges and currents on the antenna and the reactive power is radiated. Increasing the distance to the antenna (Fresnel distance R_{nf}), the radiation fields (Fresnel zone) begin but still depend on the distance to the antenna. At a certain distance away from the antenna, the radiated E-fields and H-fields are not affected by the charges and currents. This range is called far-field (Fraunhofer zone) and the corresponding distance is termed as Fraunhofer distance R_{ff}. In the far-field, the radiated wave of the antenna can be considered as a plane wave. E-fields and H-fields are in phase and the antenna pattern at this region does not depend on the distance. These three different ranges can be determined by the dimension of the antenna D_{A} and wavelength λ_{m} as follows:

$$\text{Reactive near-field:} \qquad r_{\mathrm{A}} \leq \frac{\lambda_{\mathrm{m}}}{2\pi}, \tag{3.7}$$

$$\text{Radiating near-field:} \qquad \frac{\lambda_{\mathrm{m}}}{2\pi} \leq r_{\mathrm{A}} \leq \frac{2D_{\mathrm{A}}^2}{\lambda_{\mathrm{m}}}, \tag{3.8}$$

$$\text{Far-field:} \qquad r_{\mathrm{A}} \geq \frac{2D_{\mathrm{A}}^2}{\lambda_{\mathrm{m}}}. \tag{3.9}$$

Since the human-body matched antennas are mostly operated in near-field range, the near-field antenna patterns must be characterized. In this thesis, the near-field pattern of the human-body matched antenna refers to the radiating near-field of the antenna. Since the radiation pattern is governed by the distance to the antenna, the near-field pattern must be specified for a certain distance to the antenna.

Polarization

As discussed in the previous section, the radiated EM waves from the antenna in the far-field consist of two orthogonal components: the electric and magnetic field vectors, which oscillate harmonically. The polarization of the EM waves describes the time varying direction and relative magnitude of the EM waves (normally referred to as the E-field).

Polarization can be classified as linear, circular or elliptical. In this thesis only linear polarization is considered. The field is linearly polarized, when the electric field vector always along a certain axis.

SAR

The Specific Absorption Rate (SAR) is a measure of the heating effect of EM waves on human tissues. There are two major methods to obtain the SAR value of a medical device. The technique which is based on equation (3.10) determines the change in temperature (ΔT) within a time period (Δt), while the measurement of the E-field intensity is based on (3.11).

$$\text{SAR} = C_\text{i} \cdot \frac{\Delta T}{\Delta t}. \tag{3.10}$$

$$\text{SAR} = \frac{|E|^2 \sigma}{\rho}. \tag{3.11}$$

The former technique has the drawback that most temperature sensors do not have the required sensitivity to promptly evaluate the minimal temperature gradient in a short exposure time, which is desired to minimize thermal diffusion effects. Therefore, the electric field measurement is preferred. The parameters required for the calculation are shown in equation (3.11), where $|E|$ is the magnitude of the RMS E-field and ρ is the mass density.

Typically, the 1 g or 10 g SAR is used, which is the averaged SAR value over a volume of a mass of 1 or 10 g tissue [Com01].

In this section, it has been discussed that the body-matched antennas can be characterized in terms of reflection coefficient, efficiency and radiation pattern. Additionally, the near-field pattern of the body-matched antennas in lossy medium and the SAR value in human tissues are of interest. More characterization methods of body-matched antennas (i.e. penetration efficiency and front-to-back ratio) will be discussed together with antenna configurations in chapter 5. Regarding these antenna terms, two measurement systems for the validation of the radiation pattern are introduced in the following sections.

3.2. Measurement techniques for the characterization of body-matched antennas

Due to the presence of human tissues, the antennas cannot be characterized in free space and must instead be surrounded by the corresponding tissues. However, *In vivo* measurements of each antenna with humans are not realistic and dead tissues (such as pork and beef used to emulate the human muscle) are not representative, because the ε_r and σ of tissues changes strongly after the death. Therefore, most measurements in the literature take place *in vitro*, since the dielectric properties of different human tissues were already investigated and modeled in [GLG96a, GLG96b] (see chapter 2).

In this thesis, different tissue-simulating liquids are used for the characterization of different body-matched antennas. For the on-body matched antenna, a solution of Polyethylene Glycol (PEG) 400 and water is applied as matching liquid and introduced in the following section, while a sugar-water solution is used for implantable antennas at 2.45 GHz (see chapter 4). The PEG-water solution can approximate the dielectric properties of tissues in a wide frequency range and the sugar-water solution is suitable for narrowband operation. The impedance matching and bandwidth can be measured directly by immersing the antenna into the tissue-simulating liquid.

For the characterization of the antenna radiation pattern at a short distance, an E-field probe based antenna measurement system has been developed. A 2D planar near-field antenna measurement is introduced to obtain the far-field pattern of the body-matched antennas by applying the NF-FF transformation. Since there is no standard antenna available to be immersed in a tissue-simulating liquid for the measurement, on-body matched antennas, which will be introduced in chapter 5, will be used for the measurement verification of the radiation pattern.

3.2.1. E-field probe based antenna measurement system

Since the body-matched antennas are directly in contact with human body hence has a short distance (in cm range) to the target inside the tissues, the radiation pattern of the antennas at a short distance must be investigated. However, the measurement distance is limited in the range from 40 mm (due to the geometric limitation of the antenna) to 60 mm (due to the high signal attenuation in liquid). At most frequencies, this distance corresponds to the near-field range of the antennas. For some extremely small antennas with wideband characteristic, it must be emphasized that this distance is in the far-field range at low frequencies and near-field range for high frequencies. The measurement system is characterized from 0.5 to 8 GHz with radiation pattern measurement both in the E-plane and H-plane of the antennas.

Tissue-simulating liquid

To verify the antennas in the measurement with regard to the impedance matching and radiation pattern, a tissue-simulating liquid is used to replace the human body. For the verification of the on-body matched antennas, a solution is composed of distilled water and Polyethylene Glycol (PEG) 400. The characteristics of the sugar-water solution for implantable antennas will be given in chapter 4.

PEG is a transparent liquid and is soluble in water. The different dielectric properties of the solution based on different weight ratios of distilled water and PEG are measured by a dielectric probe (85070E, Agilent) and shown in Figure 3.3. The solution can emulate tissues such as fat, skin and muscle of different permittivities. Since the on-body matched antennas are directly in contact with the human body, an averaged dielectric property of skin and fat (shown in Figure 3.3) is used to approximate the dielectric property of the human body. It can be observed in Figure 3.3 that the solution of PEG and distilled water (weight ratio of 6:4) has very similar relative permittivity to the arithmetic mean of relative permittivity of human skin and fat (averaged tissue) [GGC96]. Therefore, the 60% PEG-water solution is used to characterize the on-body matched antennas for medical diagnosis (see in chapter 5) [Sam12].

Furthermore, the signal attenuation constant versus frequency of the solution in Figure 3.4 shows that the pure PEG liquid has a very low attenuation constant. By mixing it with distilled water, the attenuation constant of the PEG-water solution increases significantly due to the increased intensity of water

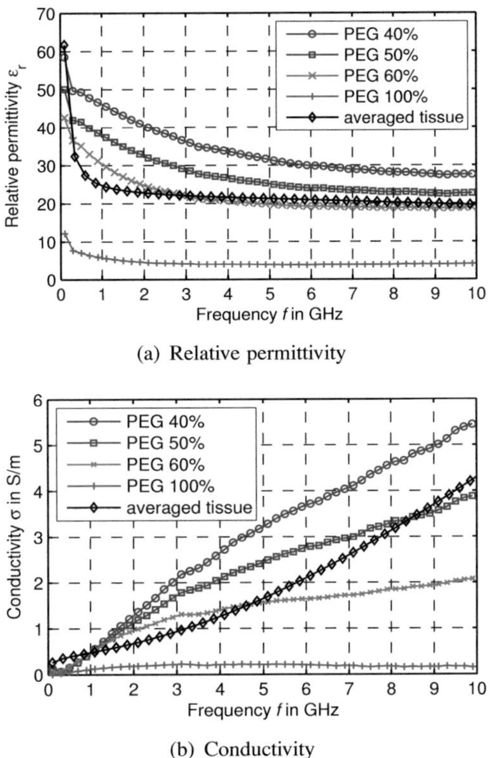

(a) Relative permittivity

(b) Conductivity

Figure 3.3.: Measured relative permittivity and conductivity of the PEG-water solutions with different water content over frequency (averaged tissue: averaged dielectric property of skin and fat predicted by Cole-Cole equation).

dipoles and the related polarization process, which can also be observed in the increasing conductivity resulting in attenuation. Moreover, the solutions indicate a slight difference of their attenuation constant in the frequency range from 1 to 3 GHz, while a large difference is present at high frequencies. In addition, the 60% solution indicates 5.8 dB/cm attenuation constant at 5 GHz, which results in a 23.2 dB attenuation at this frequency at the distance of

40 mm between the two antennas. Compared to the attenuation constant of averaged tissue, 60% PEG-water solution has similar value in the frequency range from 1 to 6 GHz, however the difference increase over the frequency up 6 GHz. In conclusion, the large relative permittivity of the liquid is obtained by mixing the PEG and water at the expense of a high signal attenuation constant, which must be tolerated in the measurement.

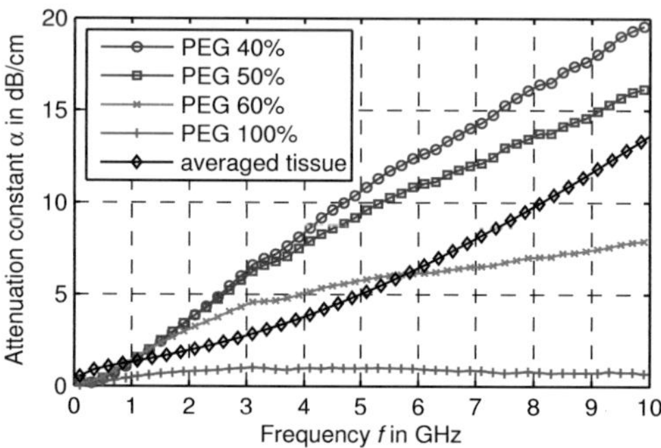

Figure 3.4.: Signal attenuation constant of the PEG-water solutions with different water content over frequency (averaged tissue: averaged dielectric property of skin and fat predicted by Cole-Cole equation).

Measurement setup of the E-field probe based antenna measurement system

The measurement setup is shown in Figure 3.5. All equipment such as the VNA and the motors are controlled by a laptop via USB interface. Two linear stages with step motors with an accuracy in the μm range are applied to adjust the position of the E-field probe in x and y directions. A rotary table with a step motor (M-062) serves to rotate the Antenna Under Test (AUT) for measurement of the radiation pattern, hence a 360° rotation in xz-plane can be performed.

To increase the dynamic range of the measurement system, (to counter the high signal attenuation in the liquid phantom), a power amplifier (Hittite) with an amplification of 19 dB from DC to 15 GHz is used. An additional low noise amplifier (LNA) can be used optionally at port 2. The dotted and solid lines in Figure 3.5 indicate the control signals for the devices and the RF signals, respectively.

The AUT is connected to port 1 of the VNA and the E-field probe to port 2. Since only a measurement distance of 40-60 mm can be achieved due to the high signal attenuation, the size of the probe is very critical for the accuracy of the measured radiation pattern. The effective area of the probe should be as small as possible compared to the aperture of the AUT [33]. Furthermore, the measured pattern of the antenna is specified for a certain distance, since the measured pattern is dependent on the measurement distance due to the short measurement distance (in most cases in near-field range).

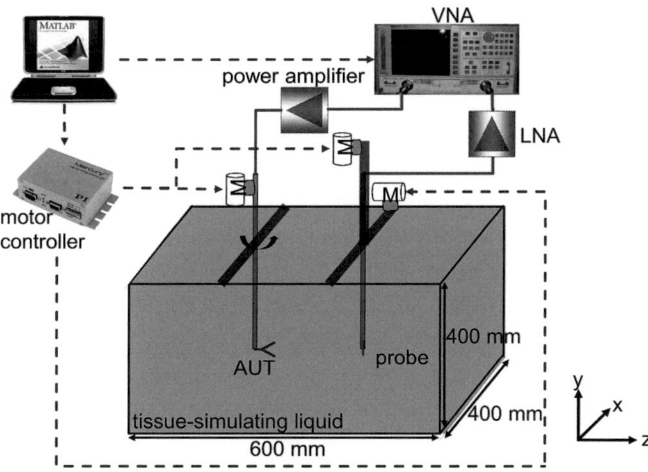

Figure 3.5.: Schematic illustration of the antenna measurement setup using tissue-simulating liquid to emulate human tissues.

An open-ended E-field probe, fabricated from a 50 Ω semi-rigid cable (5.6 mm diameter coaxial cable), is used as a coupling element in lossy medium [Smi75]. A certain length of the outer conductor and dielectric (Teflon) have been stripped off, exposing the inner conductor, as depicted in Figure 3.6

(a). The sensitivity of the probe can be improved by increasing the length or the diameter of the inner conductor [BLM06]. However the geometry of the E-field probe influences the spatial resolution as well as the accuracy of the measurement system therefore the following measurement was taken to obtain an optimal geometry. The S_{11} of the probes with different lengths of exposed inner conductor in Figure 3.6 (b) shows that the E-field probe is not matched in air but an acceptable impedance matching is achieved in PEG-water solution from 1 to 8 GHz. The S_{11} at low frequencies is improved by increasing the length of exposed inner conductor. With a longer exposed inner conductor, the probe is more sensitive to capture the radiated E-fields from AUT. However, the measurement accuracy in terms of spatial resolution can be degraded due to the large size of the probe antenna, which is comparable to the measurement distance. A length of 4 mm is used to achieve a high sensitivity of the probe, while a high accuracy of the measurement due to spatial resolution can be also provided. Its impedance matching is sufficient for capturing the E-field of the radiated wave of the AUT.

The E-field probe is inherently sensitive to the polarization of the radiated waves according to the orientation of the inner conductor. The E_y component is measured based on the configuration as shown in Figure 3.5. Therefore, the AUT can be characterized with the E-plane and H-plane patterns by rotating the AUT in the xy-plane. Since the probe is fixed during the measurement, the pattern of the probe does not effect the measurement results and an additional calibration with pattern compensation of the probe is not required. A comparison of the results between the different frequencies is extremely difficult, since the signal attenuation in the tissue-simulating liquid cannot be calculated exactly [33]. Therefore, for different frequencies, the measured S_{21} is normalized to its maximum, respectively.

The parameters of the antenna measurement system are summarized in Table 3.1. To achieve a maximum dynamic range of the measurement system, the transmitting power of the VNA is set to its maximum 5 dBm and the IF bandwidth to 100 Hz. This configuration results in a dynamic range of 100 dB. However, the frequency, at which the complete pattern in 360° of E-plane or H-plane can be measured, is still limited up to 4 GHz (at the measurement distance of 40 mm) due to the signal attenuation in PEG-water solution.

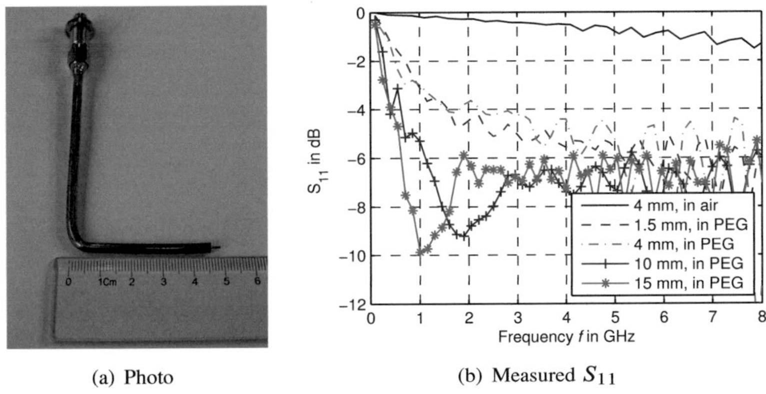

(a) Photo

(b) Measured S_{11}

Figure 3.6.: Photo and measured S_{11} of the E-field probes with different lengths of exposed inner conductor (a: photo; b: S_{11} in air and the PEG-water solution of the E-field probes with different lengths of exposed inner conductor).

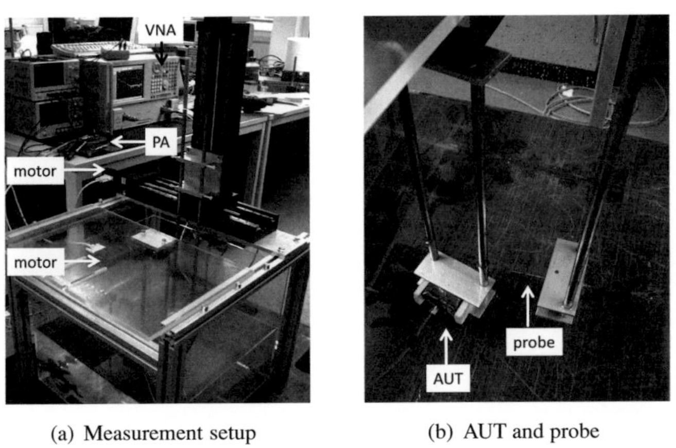

(a) Measurement setup

(b) AUT and probe

Figure 3.7.: Photos of the antenna measurement setup with tissue-simulating liquid.

Table 3.1.: Parameters of the E-field probe based antenna measurements system.

Transmitting power	5 dBm		IF bandwidth	100 Hz
Frequency range	0.5 to 4 GHz		Number of frequency points	751
Motors in use	3		Angular step	4°

A planar stepped-slot antenna optimized in the frequency range from 1 to 7 GHz [3] (the design will be explained in detail in chapter 5) is used as AUT for verification of the measurement system. For total immersion into liquid, the antenna has to be watertight so that the cavities on the top side will not be affected by the liquid as shown in Figure 3.8. Styrofoam is used to fill the cavities. The prototype is then wrapped in an absorber material with glue and copper foil to minimize the radiation to the surrounding environment. Therefore, the radiation occurs only in the half plane of the main beam direction.

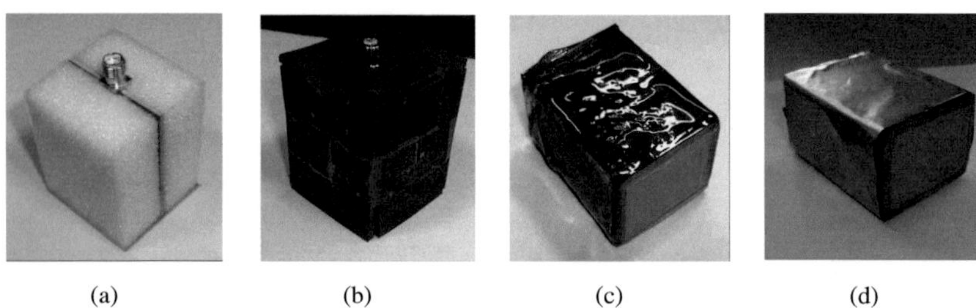

(a)   (b)   (c)   (d)

Figure 3.8.: Photos of the prototype of the stepped-slot antenna (see in chapter 5). (a: antenna with Styrofoam to maintain the free space region; b: antenna with absorber material; c: antenna with pine tar for isolation to the liquid and d: antenna with copper foil).

Verification of the E-field probe based antenna measurement system

To evaluate the performance of the E-field probe based antenna measurement system, the measured radiation pattern using AUT (the planar stepped-slot antenna) will be compared with the simulated results.

The measured S_{21} in main beam direction between the AUT and the probe at different distances are shown in Figure 3.9. In the measured S_{21}, the influence of the cable and the power amplifier are eliminated, however, the attenuation caused in the PEG-water solution is still included. The signal attenuation increases strongly versus frequency. At a distance of 20 mm, the AUT cannot be rotated completely in 360° due to the dimension of the AUT. Therefore, a distance of 40 mm was chosen, so that the measured E-field is in the radiating near-field for this antenna and the radiation pattern in 360° up to 4 GHz can be obtained completely. The S_{21} of the co-polarization (co-pol) and the cross-polarization (x-pol) at the distance of 40 mm show that the probe guarantees a polarization suppression of more than 20 dB.

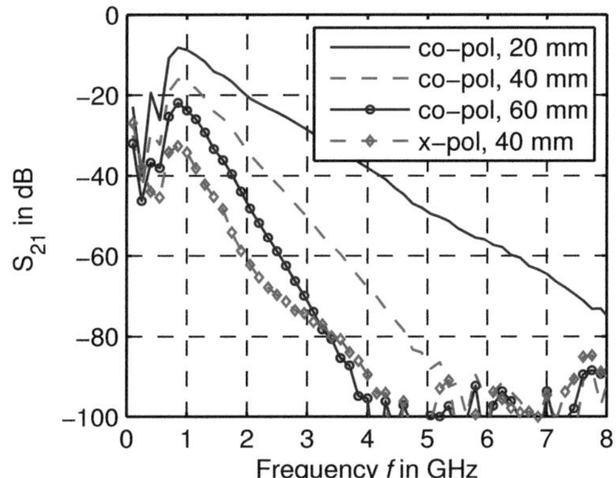

Figure 3.9.: Measured S_{21} at different distances between AUT and probe (main beam direction).

Figure 3.10 (a) and (b) show the simulated normalized pattern of the planar stepped-slot antenna at a distance of 40 mm from the antenna immersed in

PEG-water solution. This distance corresponds to the thicknesses of fat and muscle tissues of the human abdomen. Since the simulated radiation pattern up to higher frequencies (noise is not considered in CST simulation) can be obtained, the results range from 1 to 9 GHz. In the E-plane, the main beam direction is constant over the whole frequency range due to the very stable phase center. The beamwidth of the radiated E-field however decreases with frequency. At 6 and 9 GHz, two sidelobes are observed. In the H-plane, variation of main beam direction over the frequency is observed. The beam is significantly wider than the beam in the E-plane.

The measured normalized patterns of the planar stepped-slot antenna at different frequencies are shown in Figure 3.10 (c) and (d). The results are limited to 4 GHz due to the high signal attenuation in PEG solution at the higher frequencies. The measured patterns at 1 and 3 GHz both in the E-plane and H-plane are similar compared to the simulated results. The measured pattern in the H-plane with a wide beamwidth is relatively constant over the frequency. Side lobes in the E-plane are observed. The slight asymmetry of the pattern in the E-field is caused by the slightly asymmetric connection of antenna element and feed network. The difference between simulated and measured results are mostly caused by the different boundary conditions. In the simulation, the boundary is set to be an ideal open boundary without reflections. The volume of the tissue-simulating liquid in the measurement however is limited and thus the tank has only a dimension of $40 \times 60 \times 20\,\mathrm{cm}^3$. Weak reflections at the boundary of the tank contributes to the difference. The reflection from the surface of the tank at the low frequencies is of significance due to relatively low signal attenuation. Another reason could be the water leakage into the antenna (details see chapter 5).

In conclusion, the agreement between simulated and measured results confirms that the E-field probe based near-field measurement system can be used for the verification of designed body-matched antennas in terms of impedance matching and radiation pattern.

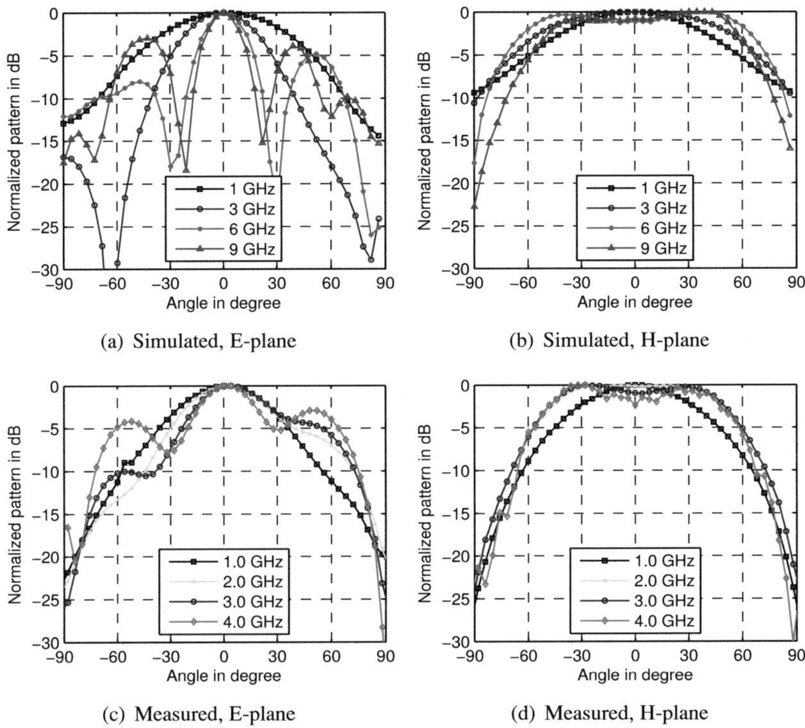

Figure 3.10.: Simulated and measured normalized radiation pattern of the planar stepped-slot antenna in the E-plane and H-plane at a distance of 40 mm.

3.2.2. Planar-rectangular near-field measurement system

Though the body-matched antennas are used for near-field range operation, the far-field pattern and gain of the antennas can be characterized as a measure of the antenna performance. In simulation, the far-field pattern and gain of the antennas can easily be calculated by excluding the conductivity of the medium. In this way, the signal attenuation caused by the lossy medium is not included. However, in most cases, the pattern in the far-field cannot be measured directly, since the tissue-simulating liquid (PEG-water solution) causes a high signal attenuation and thus, the measurement distance is strongly limited.

To counter this limitation, a different measurement setup is required. A planar-rectangular near-field antenna measurement system is designed to obtain the far-field pattern of the body-matched antennas. The electric near-field of the AUT immersed in the PEG-water solution is measured and the far-field pattern is processed through NF-FF transformation. The principle of the NF-FF Transformation and the planar-rectangular near-field measurement system setup are provided as follows.

Principle of NF-FF Transformation

The planar NF-FF transformation is based on the plane wave spectrum approach using Fourier transform. The E-field in the far-field region can be determined by

$$\vec{E}(x,y,z) = \frac{1}{4\pi^2} \int_{-\infty}^{\infty} \int_{-\infty}^{\infty} \vec{F}(k_x,k_y)e^{-j\vec{k}\cdot\vec{r}}\,dk_x dk_y, \qquad (3.12)$$

where $\vec{F}$ is the plane wave spectrum, k_x and k_y are the wave numbers of the plane wave spectrum in x and y directions, respectively [Bal05]. $\vec{r} = \vec{r}(x,y,z)$ is the distance to the origin of the coordinate system.

In the framework of the proposed near-field antenna measurement, a planar-rectangular scanning for the acquisition of the E-field in the near-field region of the AUT is applied. According to the coordinate system for the antenna measurement setup (refer to Figure 3.12), two components of the E-fields in the x and y directions can be obtained from the measurements. Assuming that E_{x0} and E_{y0} are the measured tangential electric near-fields over the plane scanned by the beams ($z = 0$), the aforementioned plane wave spectrum (F_x and F_y in x and y directions) can be written as [Bal05] [GMP07]

$$F_x(k_x,k_y) = \int_{-\infty}^{\infty}\int_{-\infty}^{\infty} E_{x0}(x,y,z=0)e^{j(k_x x+k_y y)}dxdy, \qquad (3.13)$$

$$F_y(k_x,k_y) = \int_{-\infty}^{\infty}\int_{-\infty}^{\infty} E_{y0}(x,y,z=0)e^{j(k_x x+k_y y)}dxdy. \qquad (3.14)$$

With the known plane wave spectrum, the E-field in the far-field region can be obtained. To present far-field pattern in terms of spherical angles, the E-fields for two planes (E-plane and H-plane) can be modified to

$$E_\theta(r,\theta,\varphi) \simeq j\frac{ke^{-jkr}}{2\pi r}[F_x cos\varphi + F_y sin\varphi], \qquad (3.15)$$

$$E_\phi(r,\theta,\varphi) \simeq j\frac{ke^{-jkr}}{2\pi r}cos\theta[-F_x sin\varphi + F_y sin\varphi]. \qquad (3.16)$$

Taking the medium with high permittivity into account, the wavenumber can be written as

$$k = 2\pi f\frac{\mathrm{Re}\left\{\sqrt{\varepsilon_\mathrm{r} - j\frac{\sigma}{\omega\varepsilon_0}}\right\}}{c_0}, \qquad (3.17)$$

The imaginary part of the wave number is ignored and the signal attenuation is not considered in the transformation algorithm, since the results are normalized in spherical coordinate system at each frequency.

Moreover, in the planar-rectangular scanning, the dimension of the scan area is limited by the real size of the measurement system and the strong signal attenuation in the tissue-simulating liquid, in which the antenna is immersed. Therefore, the missing information outside the scan area limits the maximum achievable angle θ_{max} after NF-FF Transformation [GMP07]. Furthermore, the truncation error for the given size of the scanning area restricts the θ_{max} [DFG$^+$08]. The maximum achievable angle θ_{max} is illustrated in Figure 3.11 (a), where the D_{A1} and D_{A2} are the apertures of the AUT and the probe antenna in one direction (x or y), L is the length of the scan area. θ_{max} can be estimated by (3.18). In Table 3.2, different θ_{max} are provided with respect to the L and r_A (assuming the aperture of the measured antenna $D_{A1} = 35\,\text{mm}$, $D_{A1} = D_{A2}$) [Sam12].

$$\theta_{max} = \arctan\left(\frac{L - D_{A1} - D_{A2}}{2r_A}\right). \tag{3.18}$$

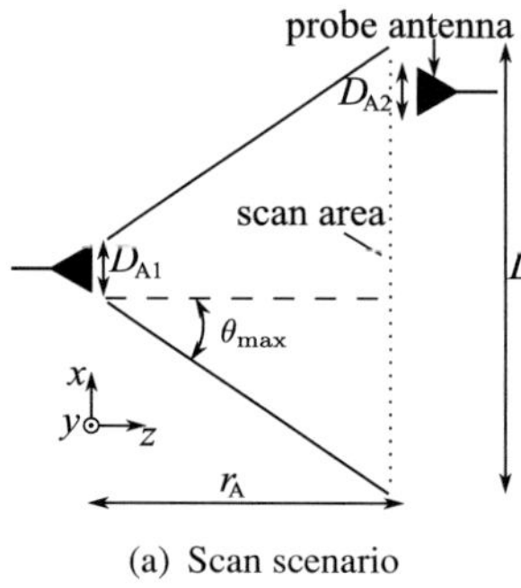

(a) Scan scenario

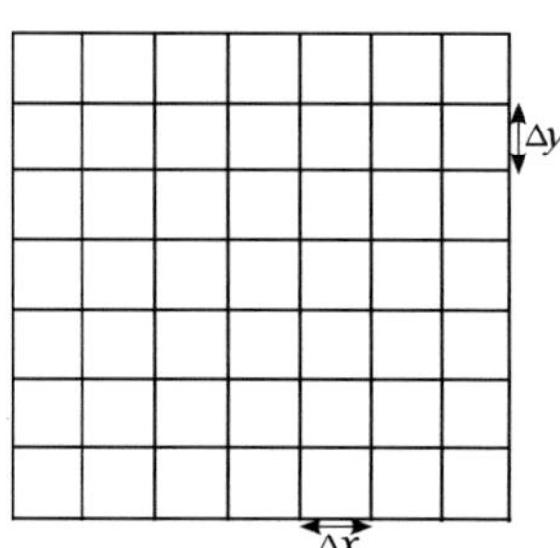

(b) Scan area (xy-plane with dotted line in (a))

Figure 3.11.: Schematic representation of the scenario for the determination of the θ_{max} and the scan area.

To achieve a large θ_{max}, a very large scan area and huge tank with PEG-water solution are required, which is difficult to be realized. Therefore, planar-rectangular scanning is more suitable for antennas with high gain and small beamwidth.

Table 3.2.: Maximum achievable angle θ_{max} in the far-field pattern depending on L and r_A.

L in mm	104	104	112	112	120	120
r_A in mm	15	20	15	20	15	20
θ_{max} in degree	48.57	40.36	54.46	46.40	59.04	51.34

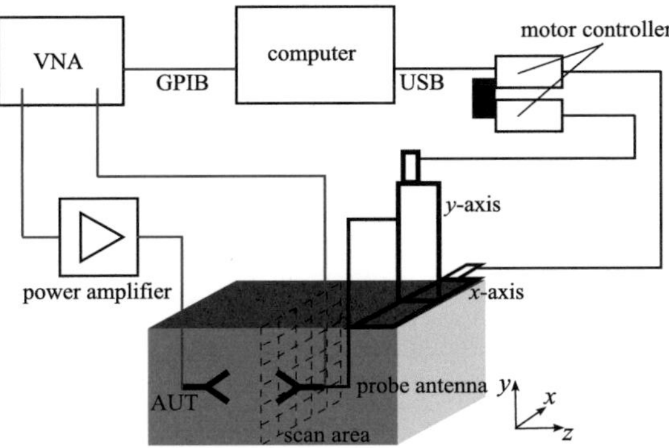

Figure 3.12.: Block diagram of the planar-rectangular near-field antenna measurement system.

Measurement setup of the planar-rectangular near-field measurement

The planar-rectangular near-field measurement system uses a similar setup as the E-field probe based measurement system and is illustrated in Figure 3.12. The design of the overall measurement system with its important parameters is given in Table 3.3. The AUT is connected to port 1 of the VNA and the probe with port 2. Two identical antennas (the planar stepped-slot antenna) are used as AUT and probe, since the antenna is required to be immersed in the liquid and traditional horn antennas or open-ended waveguide probes are not suitable. The PEG-water solution is also used as tissue-simulating liquid. The relative permittivity of the PEG-water solution is taken into account in the transformation algorithm.

Since the electric near-field is measured and the far-field pattern is obtained through a NF-FF Transformation, the near-field and far-field range must be analyzed for a certain antenna. The far-field range (Fraunhofer distance) can be calculated using (3.9), where D_A is the largest aperture of the antenna (diagonal: 43.6 mm). ε_r is the relative permittivity of the tissue-simulating liquid. As an approximation, the ε_r is assumed to be 20 for the whole frequency range from 1 to 8 GHz, which is used in the antenna design in the

Table 3.3.: Design parameters of the planar-rectangular near-field measurement system.

frequency range	0.5 - 8 GHz
frequency points	751
scan length in x direction	104 mm
scan length in y direction	104 mm
scan step in x and y direction	4 mm
measurement distance in z direction	15 mm

simulation (see chapter 5). The reactive near-field and far-field range of the antenna are given in Table 3.4. The measurement should be performed in the radiating near-field range of the antenna [32]. Regarding the R_{nf} (Fresnel distance) and the R_{ff} (Fraunhofer distance) in the frequency range from 1 to 8 GHz, a measurement distance of 15 mm between the AUT and the probe antenna is chosen.

Table 3.4.: Reactive near-field and far-field range of the measurement antenna at different frequencies based on a frequency independent $\varepsilon_{\mathrm{r}} = 20$.

f (GHz)	1	3	5	7	8
R_{nf} (mm)	10.68	3.56	2.13	1.53	1.34
R_{ff} (mm)	56.67	170.03	283.52	396.03	453.15

Moreover, the scan steps in the x (Δx) and the y (Δy) direction both are chosen to be 4 mm so that a maximum uniform sample spacing $\lambda_{\mathrm{m}}/2$ is maintained. The scanning area is set to be $104 \times 104\,\mathrm{mm}^2$. A planar stepped-slot antenna with a size of $26 \times 35\,\mathrm{mm}^2$ is used as AUT for the antenna measurement. This configuration results in maximum achievable angles of $60°$ and $48.6°$ in the E-plane and H-plane, respectively.

Verification of the planar-rectangular near-field measurement

For the NF-FF Transformation, the E-fields in both the co- and cross-polarization of the AUT are required. The measured raw data at different frequencies are shown in Figure 3.13. Since the maximum magnitude of S_{21} in Co-polarization decreases strongly with the frequency due to the increase of the signal attenuation over frequency, the near-field pattern is normalized at each frequency, respectively. Moreover, for a better comparison between co- and cross-polarization, the magnitude of S_{21} is normalized to the maximum of co-polarization at each frequency.

It can be observed that at 1 GHz the maximum magnitude of S_{21} in co-polarization is normalized to be 0 dB, where the receiving antenna is placed in the center of the scan zone. On the edge of the scan area, the S_{21} drops to -49 dB. However, the measurement in cross-polarization indicates -30 dB of S_{21} in the center of the scan area and the value increases to a maximum (-15 dB) at (x=12 mm, y=12 mm). At 1 and 4 GHz, 4 maximums can be seen in cross-polarization. Moreover, these results show that the AUT exhibits a very good cross-polarization suppression [32].

Furthermore, the raw data at the lower frequencies show a wider beamwidth than at the higher frequencies, which must result in a wide pattern in far-field at the low frequencies after NF-FF transformation. This agrees with the theoretical analysis that at the low frequencies the antenna provides a wide pattern due to the small electrical dimensions of the antenna.

In Figure 3.14, the normalized patterns processed by the NF-FF transformation are provided in the E-plane and H-plane. The results are compared with the simulated pattern at different frequencies. In simulation, the dielectric property of the PEG-water solution is also implemented. The scan area, scan step and antenna distance remain as in the measurement setup for the verification.

It can be seen that the far-field radiation pattern at the higher frequencies (i.e. 6 and 8 GHz) could also be obtained using this planar-rectangular near-field antenna measurement system and NF-FF transformation, which cannot be measured directly in the E-field probe based measurement system due to the extreme high signal attenuation (in the far-field range). The processed far-field patterns based on the simulated and measured data agree with each other at 1 and 4 GHz. At 6 and 8 GHz, differences between simulated and measured results are observed, which are caused by the different boundaries of the lossy medium in the simulation and measurement. However, a remarkable similar-

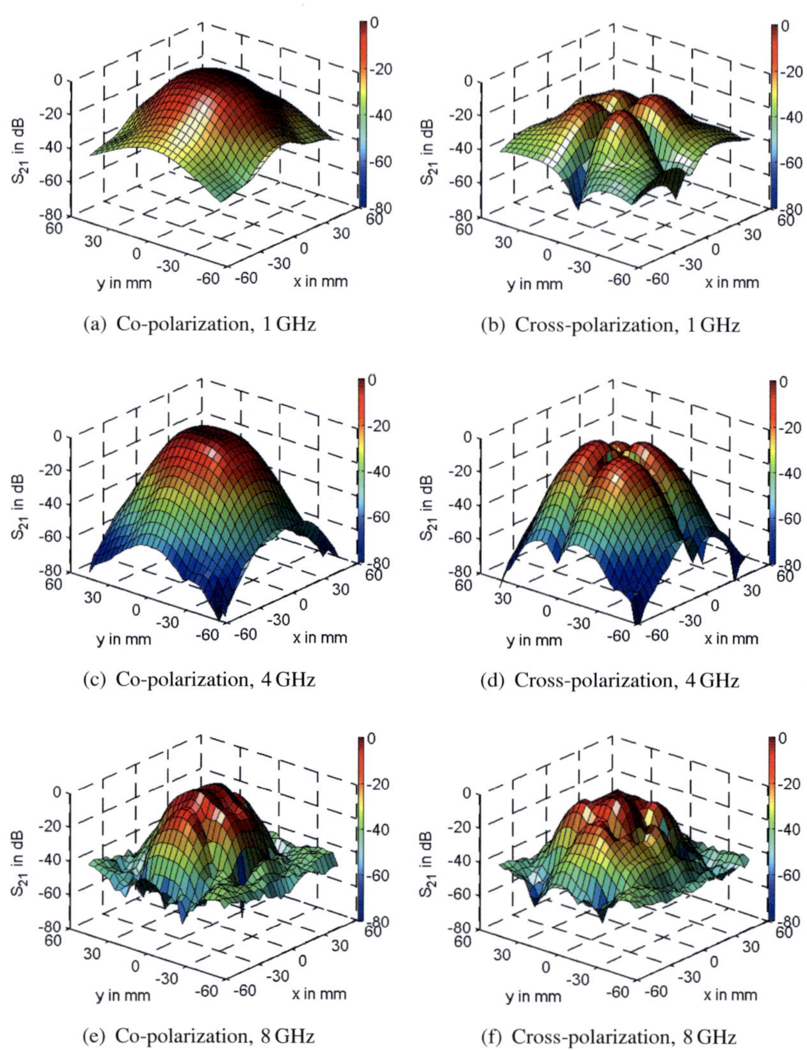

(a) Co-polarization, 1 GHz

(b) Cross-polarization, 1 GHz

(c) Co-polarization, 4 GHz

(d) Cross-polarization, 4 GHz

(e) Co-polarization, 8 GHz

(f) Cross-polarization, 8 GHz

Figure 3.13.: Measured raw data S_{21} at different frequencies over the whole scan area: (a) in co-ploarization and (b) in cross-polarization.

ity of the pattern can be confirmed. In conclusion, the planar-rectangular near-field antenna measurement system enables to verify the far-field radiation pattern of the body-matched antennas.

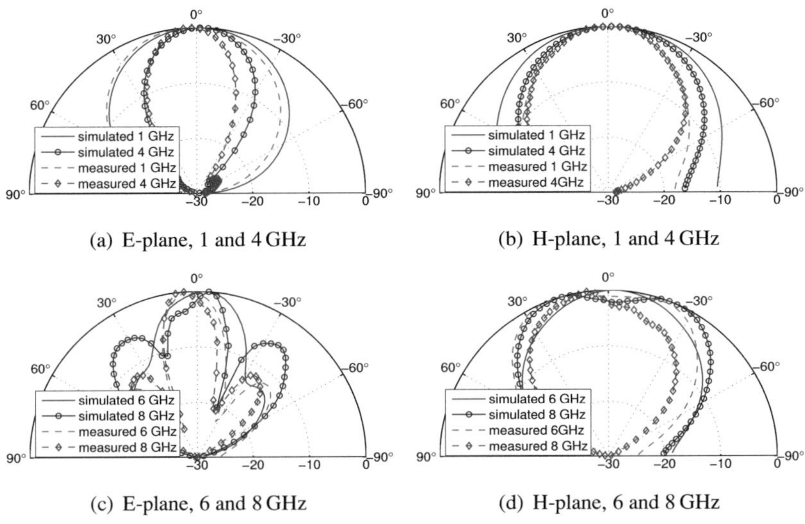

(a) E-plane, 1 and 4 GHz

(b) H-plane, 1 and 4 GHz

(c) E-plane, 6 and 8 GHz

(d) H-plane, 6 and 8 GHz

Figure 3.14.: Far-field patterns obtained using the NF-FF transformation of simulated and measured data at different frequencies in the E-plane and H-plane, co-polarization (normalized in dB).

3.3. Summary

Different characterization methods for the evaluation of the body-matched antennas have been discussed in this chapter. The body-matched antennas can be characterized like the antennas for free-space operation in terms of impedance matching, antenna gain and radiation efficiency. Regarding the radiation pattern, the near-field and far-field patterns can be used. For the body-matched antenna, in particular the near-field pattern is of significance, since the body-matched antennas are used at a short distance to the target. In addition, the SAR value is a special characteristic of antennas for medical applications and required to be evaluated to guarantee the safety for the human body with regard to the RF radiation.

To verify the characteristics such as impedance matching and radiation pattern of the body-matched antennas, two special antenna measurement systems are developed: the E-field probe based measurement system and the planar-rectangular near-field measurement system. To approximate the dielectric properties of human tissues (surrounding medium of body-matched antennas) in the measurement, tissue-simulating liquid (PEG-water solution) is used. The body-matched antennas must be immersed into the liquid in the measurement. The results show that the E-field probe based antenna measurement system enables a measurement of the radiation pattern at a short distance to the body-matched antennas. However, the measurement distance is limited (40-60 mm) in terms of SNR of the received signal due to the high signal attenuation in tissue-simulating liquid. To obtain the far-field pattern of the antennas, the planar-rectangular near-field measurement system is applied to measure the electric near-fields. Then the far-field pattern is obtained by using a NF-FF transformation. The verified results (compared to the simulation results) confirm that these measurement systems are feasible to measure the radiation far-field pattern of the body-matched antennas in the E- and H-plane. In the following chapters, the emphasis will be on the near-field pattern of these antennas, since the antennas will be operated at a short distance. Therefore, the E-field probe based antenna measurement system will be used for the verification of the to-be-designed antennas.

After considering the characterization methods of body-matched antennas and the development of the measurement systems, the implantable antennas for data telemetry and on-body matched antennas for medical diagnosis will be introduced in the following two chapters.

4. Implantable antennas for wireless communication of IMDs

This chapter deals with one of the major microwave applications in the medical field: data transmission between implanted and external devices. Based on this application, this chapter focuses on the design of implantable antennas in terms of their small size, high efficiency and robust performance. First, an overview of the state-of-art research and challenges for the wireless communication of the IMDs are given. Based on these challenges and requirements for the implantable antennas, the design of the stripline-fed double-layer slot antennas is then provided together with miniaturization techniques to optimize the antenna structures. The proposed antennas are intended to be implanted in the muscle tissues in the human body. The simulation results are validated in the measurement using sugar-water solution, which emulates the muscle tissues. This chapter is concluded with a performance comparison of the three antennas with regard to their bandwidth, size, efficiency and sensitivity against permittivity variation of the muscle tissues.

4.1. Overview of wireless communication of IMDs

For most modern IMDs, using a wireless communication link between implants and external devices is the optimum choice compared to using wired connection. Contrary to traditional methods of using wires for the connection with the implanted devices for the acquisition of diagnosis signals, implants based on wireless communication require minimum incision into the body. Inspections of IMDs can be then carried out without frequent chirurgical operation. Wireless communication of IMDs enables the reduction of costs (e.g.

maintenance cost of devices), lowers the risk of infection due to the wires, which leads to the increase of comfort for the patients. Furthermore, such telemetry systems of IMDs have the possibility of monitoring the patient's physical state as well as controlling the functionalities of the devices at a certain distance between the external devices and the patient. The data can then be transfered immediately to the medical center. In emergency situations, it allows the immediate detection and treatment of physical abnormalities, which results in time saving and eliminating hospitalization costs by home care monitoring [SSC94].

To limit the radiation of RF devices and to guarantee a safe level of human exposure to RF emissions, regulations are set up by the Federal Communications Commission (FCC) with regard to the operational frequency bands and power limitations, which will be discussed in the following sections. Then, the challenges of wireless performance for IMDs will be described.

4.1.1. Frequency bands and power limitations

Wireless IMDs are allowed to operate in several frequency bands according to the different standards in different countries. Depending on the data rate, operational distance and power transfer capability, different radiation regulations are applied. The FCC has distributed the spectrum allocations shown in Table 4.1 for medical applications [Com01, Ser09, ITU01].

Table 4.1.: Frequency bands and power limitations for medical devices according to the FCC.

Band	Frequency	Maximum EIRP
MedRadio	401-406 MHz	-16 dBm
ISM	2.4-2.5 GHz	20 dBm

As established by the FCC, the operational frequency bands for medical applications are mainly the Medical Device Radiocommunications Service (MedRadio) from 401 MHz to 406 MHz and the Industrial, Scientific and Medical Radio (ISM) band from 2.4 to 2.5 GHz. The MedRadio band is used by a variety of devices in and near the human body to extend the previously established

Medical Implant Communication Service (MICS), which mostly comprises communication of IMDs. This band is preferred where low interference is required. However, the ISM Band has the advantage of smaller achievable antenna size due to shorter wavelength and authorization of unlicensed use. Furthermore, these medical devices have to adhere to the power limitation set by the FCC in Table 4.1 to minimize the interference to other existing RF systems. This is also due to the impact of EM fields on human tissues, which causes hazardous dielectric heating. This then leads to tissue burns and disturbance to the human body functionality caused by the rise of the temperature as well as blood pressure [oNiRPI98]. The heating effect can be quantitatively determined in terms of SAR. The International Commission on Non-Ionizing Radiation Protection (ICNIRP) has established the European limit for SAR of 2 W/kg averaged over 10 g of tissues. In the United States the requirements are stricter, as the FCC allows a maximum power of 1.6 W/kg averaged over 1 g of tissues.

With the limitations of frequency bands and radiation power of the IMDs in mind, the main challenges of telemetry systems with IMDs come down to the design of implantable antennas, which is the focus of this chapter. A well designed implantable antenna should be light, small yet fulfills the technical requirements of efficient RF radiation and transmission. The design of small-sized implantable antennas in the ISM band is considered, which allows a miniaturization of the implants. The details about the challenges of the antenna design can be found in the following section.

4.1.2. Challenges of the implantable antenna design

The implantable antennas should fulfill various requirements such as having a high efficiency, stable pattern and low SAR value. The high radiation efficiency in turn contributes to the low energy consumption of the overall implants and therefore a long operating time of the battery, which then reduces the times of changing the battery by means of chirurgical operation. SAR is related to the exposure of the human tissues to RF. A low SAR value means a low exposure to RF. Therefore the SAR value is capped at a maximum allowable safe value for RF medical devices. The SAR distribution is also dependent on the geometrical model of the human body and the radiation pattern of the implantable antenna. Therefore, highly directional radiation pattern of the implantable antenna must be prevented and an omni-directional pattern is desirable.

Another challenge is that the radiation performance of the implantable antennas is dependent on the location in the body, where it is embedded. Since the implantable antennas are totally surrounded by human tissues, the characteristics of the implantable antennas such as resonance frequency, bandwidth, efficiency and input impedance are strongly dependent on the dielectric properties of the surrounding tissues. Most of the implantable antennas are designed using a resonant structure with narrow bandwidth. The problem with using a resonant structure is that the shift of the resonance frequency of the antenna due to the change of the relative permittivity of the surrounding tissues (change of water content of tissues or difference between different individuals), causes significant degradation of the performance of the devices (e.g. efficiency). The reduced efficiency results in a short battery lifetime of IMDs. Furthermore, the radiating element usually must be electrically isolated to prevent a short circuit by ions in the tissue. Requirements for the coating materials used include bio-compatibility, mechanical robustness and long-term durability. In conclusion, the robustness of the antenna in terms of impedance matching and radiation efficiency is extremely important, which should be validated in a realistic scenario.

For the verification of the antenna performance, *in vivo* measurements on humans are difficult to be permitted, whereas measurements carried out on live test subjects (e.g. rats) are expensive. Therefore, *in vitro* measurements are often applied, where only slight differences are observed in comparison with the *in vivo* measurements [GLG96a]. As the ε_r and σ of tissues change significantly after death, fresh meat such as beef and pork cannot be used as the phantom. Currently, liquid phantoms are preferred to emulate the dielectric property of human tissues for implantable antennas due to their high stability of the dielectric property and low cost.

For implantable antennas, it is desirable that the size is as small as possible to minimize the site of implantation. Since the size of an antenna is directly proportional to the operating wavelength, further miniaturization techniques must be employed. Therefore different methods for miniaturization have been addressed in the literature. For devices to be placed between skin and muscle, for instance, a shorted pin on a spiral structure to the ground is introduced [KRS04]. A smaller size of the proposed antenna was achieved compared to the microstrip antenna. A four layer stacked triple band antenna was introduced in [HLC$^+$11]. The electric path of the surface current has been lengthened by the design of a meandered structure in [KHT08] and the antenna size was significantly reduced. However, the antenna suffers from a limited bandwidth of several tens of MHz. Moreover, a lower radiation efficiency of the many implantable antennas have to be tolerated.

The goal of this chapter is to design a miniaturized implantable antenna with a high efficiency, omni-directional radiation properties and robust performance with the slight changing of the dielectric properties of tissues. To be able to design a small-sized antenna, the ISM band (2.4 to 2.5 GHz) is chosen instead of the MedRadio band. For the operation of the antenna in the ISM band, the antenna must have a bandwidth larger than 100 MHz. In the following section, the details of the design principles will be given.

4.2. Design of stripline-fed double-layer slot antennas

First of all, the location of the implantable antenna becomes critical for the antenna design, since the implantable antennas are completely surrounded by human tissues. Table 4.2 shows the dielectric properties of different tissues at the ISM band (2.45 GHz). The relative permittivity of blood, liver and muscle are very similar, while a large difference between fat and muscle is observed. Thus, the location of the implantable antennas must be determined at first.

It can be found that a large number of common implanted devices such as pacemakers, defibrillators, and radio-frequency identification (RFID) implants are located in the muscle tissues. Therefore, the main objective of this chapter is to design implantable antennas, which can be embedded in or between the muscle tissues. It is desirable that the antenna has an omnidirectional pattern so that signals can be sent to the base station (external devices) regardless of the patient's orientation towards the base station.

Table 4.2.: Dielectric properties of human tissues at 2.45 GHz [GGC96, GLG96a].

Tissue	ε_r	σ in S/m
Blood	58.26	2.545
Heart	54.81	2.256
Muscle	52.72	1.73
Liver	43.03	1.686
Fat	5.28	0.104

In the literature, several designs of implantable antennas with a three dimensional structure are addressed in [MBZ$^+$11]. In [WSTI09], an implanted three-dimensional H-shaped cavity slot antenna is proposed for short range wireless communications. However, a high fabrication complexity is associated with it. To reduce the fabrication complexity and cost of implantable antennas, antenna designs with planar structures are considered in this thesis. Regarding the feeding technique of the implantable antenna, a stripline-fed technique is used instead of a microstrip feed to minimize the spurious radiation (e.g. leaky waves) along the feed line, which is surrounded by the muscle tissues with a high relative permittivity. This is because the microstrip feeding line leads to an additional loss thus causing undesired reduction of the total radiation efficiency. Figure 4.1 illustrates the E-field distributions of microstrip and stripline in the muscle tissues. Figure 4.1 (a) shows the microstrip located between the substrate ($\varepsilon_{r,sub}$= 10.2) and muscle (ε_r= 52.72), which results in strong surface and leaky waves. The surface waves are partly absorbed in the muscle tissues, while the leaky waves cause the distortion of the radiation pattern. Therefore, the realized gain and efficiency of the implantable antenna will be severely reduced. Moreover, the wave impedance of the microstrip line changes, hence the impedance matching at the antenna port is degraded, with the change of the dielectric properties of the muscle tissues (change of the water content of different individuals). The antenna fed by slotline and coplanar waveguide (CPW) suffers from the same problem in the design of implantable antennas [SFC04].

In the case of a stripline configuration as shown in Figure 4.1 (b), the feed is enclosed by two ground planes. No surface or leaky waves occur and hence the crosstalk to the muscle tissues is prevented, i.e. no distortion of the radiation pattern is introduced by the feed line. Furthermore, the wave impedance of the stripline is independent of the dielectric property of the surrounding tissues, since the electric fields are totally enclosed between the two ground planes. This results in the elimination of dispersion and the propagation of pure transverse electromagnetic (TEM) waves.

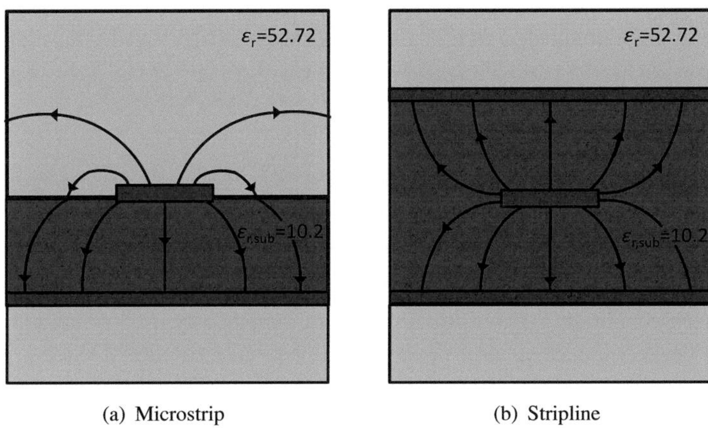

(a) Microstrip   (b) Stripline

Figure 4.1.: Schematic illustration of the E-field distributions of microstrip (a) and stripline (b) between the substrate ($\varepsilon_{r,sub}$= 10.2) and muscle tissues (ε_r= 52.72).

For a size reduction of the antenna, a simple method is to increase the relative permittivity ε_r and the thickness h_s of the substrate. However, the increase of $\varepsilon_{r,sub}$ decreases the achievable bandwidth [KKYP01]. With increasing h_s, fringing fields are enforced, leading to extension of the electric field lines over the actual antenna geometry. The antenna appears electrically larger, resulting in a shift of resonance frequency into the lower frequency range. However, for large h_s, the surface waves dominate. A part of the input power is converted in surface waves instead of being radiated. In addition, reflection and scattering at the substrate's physical boundaries increase the cross-polarization level, thus reducing the gain and the radiation efficiency. Also, the radiation pattern is distorted. Therefore, ε_r and h_s must be chosen carefully.

Another technique for size reduction is to increase the electrical length of the radiator by introducing slots or fractal structures. Two planar implantable antennas with meandered strips have been presented in [KHT08] and [KRS06]. In [KKYP01] the rectangular stripline-fed meandered slot antenna is investigated. A significant reduction of the size of the antenna is obtained. However, the antenna features a very narrow band. A slight frequency shift caused by the change of the dielectric properties of tissues lead to the impedance mismatch of the antenna and thus a reduced antenna efficiency. In this chapter, a slot antenna combined with a meandered structure is proposed to maintain a certain bandwidth of the antenna and to reduce the antenna size at the same time.

In the following sections, three different stripline-fed slot antennas are introduced with the consideration of the challenges and problems mentioned in section 4.1.2. The antennas are designed and characterized at the ISM band. Among these antennas, the basic model is the antenna with equal-sized meandered strips. The size of this antenna is then reduced by optimizing the shape of the meandered strips and the ground, respectively, which results in two miniaturized antennas. All three antennas are validated in the measurements and discussed in the final section of this chapter.

4.2.1. Stripline-fed slot antenna with equally-sized meandered strips (M3-1)

The implantable antenna (M3-1) comprises two planar layers with the same substrate. The three structures of the antenna (top side, bottom side and radiator between the two substrates) are shown in Figure 4.2. The rectangular slots (Structure 2) at the top and the bottom are ground planes with the same structure. Structure 1 consists of meandered strips connected with the stripline of 50 Ω line impedance.

Benefiting from the meandered radiator, the size of the antenna is reduced, since the electrical length of the structure is increased. The slotted grounds at the top and bottom side enable a large bandwidth [39]. After the investigation

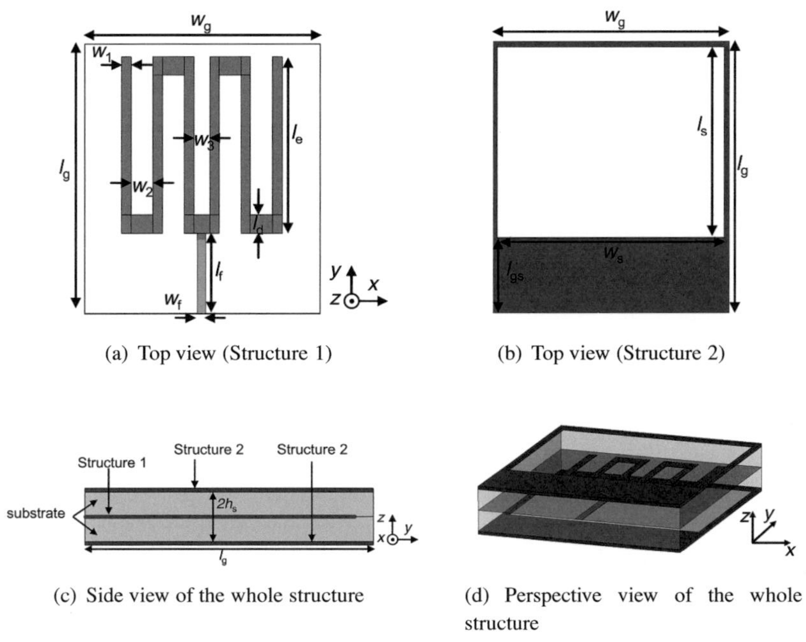

Figure 4.2.: Layout of the antenna M3-1 (Grey color denotes the metal).

of several designs of meandered strips with regard to the inductive behavior and mutual coupling between meandered strips, three-armed meandered strips show the best performance with respect to the impedance matching and size reduction of the whole antenna. The radiation efficiency of the antenna is increased by using a stripline feed to prevent the radiation along the feed line (as discussed in the last section). The three dimensional (3D) view of the double-layer slot antenna is shown in Figure 4.2 (d). The substrate Rogers RT 6010 with the dielectric constant of 10.2, $\tan\delta$ of 0.0023 and thickness of 1.27 mm is chosen for the antenna design and fabrication.

With regard to the meandered strips, the excitation mode is equivalent to that of a stub antenna with the same length as a straight elongated meandered strip. As can be deduced from the alignment of the surface current vectors in the simulation, the antenna in Figure 4.2 excites a resonance of $\frac{3}{4}$ wavelength at 2.45 GHz. The effective electrical length of the meandered strips can be calculated by

$$L_{sp} = k_{sp}\lambda = k_{sp} \cdot \frac{c_0}{\sqrt{\varepsilon_{r,\text{eff}}} \cdot f}, \tag{4.1}$$

where k_{sp} is the fraction of the resonant wavelength (in this case is $\frac{3}{4}$) and f is the resonance frequency. The real electrical length of the meandered strips is slightly different from the predicted one, since the parasitic effects between the strips must be taken into account. The lumped circuit model shown in Figure 4.3 aids the comprehension of the meandered antenna's non-ideal electric behavior [ESSK00]. In this model, each strip is represented by the inductance of its magnetic field. The magnetic field lines rotate around the metallic strips. At the edges of meandered strips charges accumulate to induce a capacitive effect. Cascading each meandered segment results in the final equivalent circuit. The open ended meandered strip is represented by capacitances in order to model the fringing fields with the substrate. As the structure is symmetrical to the xy-plane, Figure 4.3 depicts one half of the equivalent circuit.

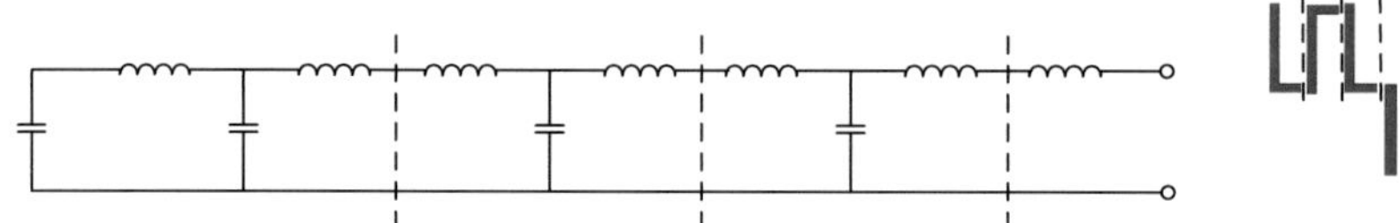

Figure 4.3.: Equivalent lumped circuit model of the antenna M3-1 with capacitances and inductances.

Since the antenna is implanted in the human muscle, in simulation, a muscle phantom (ε_r=52.72, σ=1.73 S/m) emulating the dielectric property of real muscle tissues is used (dielectric property as muscle at 2.45 GHz).

At first, the antenna parameters are optimized without considering the conductivity of the phantom, since then the radiation pattern and efficiency can be observed without signal attenuation caused by the lossy phantom. Therefore, only the relative permittivity (ε_r=52.72) is applied in the simulation. After the first optimization step without the loss of the phantom, this loss is then added, to observe its impact on the designed antenna.

The resonance frequency of the slot antenna is related to the size of the slot (l_s and w_s), on which the size of whole antenna is dependent. Furthermore, by optimizing the parameters of the meandered strips, the resonance frequency can be also decreased. Therefore, the size of the slot can be reduced by introducing the meandered strips while the resonance frequency is maintained. Furthermore, increasing the length of the meandered strips l_e and decreasing l_d leads to a low resonance frequency, since the electrical length of meandered strips is elongated. Moreover, the simulation results show that a large w_2 leads to a low resonance frequency. Since the coupling within the meandered strips is reduced by their increased distance (w_2), the electrical length of the strips is hence increased. The impedance matching becomes also better and a strong resonance is obtained. However, the bandwidth is slightly reduced. Therefore, a compromise has to be made between the resonance frequency and bandwidth. The resonance frequency of the antenna shifts according to the change of the dielectric properties of the muscle tissues (different individuals). Therefore, a large bandwidth of the antenna enables the robustness of the impedance matching (to be under -10 dB) of the implantable antenna at the ISM band despite of a slight shift of the resonance frequency.

Observing the current distribution of the antenna in the simulation, the ground size (w_g, l_g and the thickness of the slot edge) can be reduced without significant modification to the antenna characteristics, since the strong surface current is concentrated around the slot edge.

A semi-rigid coaxial cable (Farnell, RG402U) is used, which has an inner diameter of 0.9 mm and an outer diameter of 3.58 mm, as the antenna feed. The simulation result in Figure 4.4 (a) shows that the antenna fed by the coaxial cable with a length of 5 cm has a similar impedance matching with the one fed by a waveguide port in CST.

Now that the antenna characteristics have been determined, the conductivity of muscle tissue (σ=1.73 S/m) is considered in the simulation to include the losses caused by the phantom. From the result in Figure 4.4 (b), the change of S_{11} and the resonance frequency is indistinguishable. Therefore, only a slight optimization of some parameters is required to obtain a resonance frequency at 2.45 GHz.

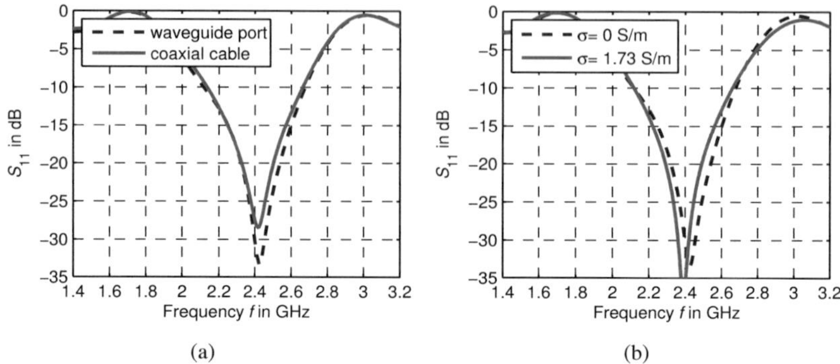

Figure 4.4.: Simulated influences of excitation port (a) and conductivity of surrounding tissue (b) in reflection coefficient of the stripline-fed slot antenna (M3-1).

After the optimization procedure of all parameters, the final optimized parameters are given in Table 4.3. The M3-1 antenna has an overall size of $14.5 \times 12.5 \times 2.54\,\mathrm{mm}^3$. The final version of this antenna has a relative bandwidth of 19.5%, ranging from 2.16 to 2.68 GHz in simulation.

Table 4.3.: Parameters of the antenna M3-1.

Parameters	w_g	l_g	l_{gs}	w_s	l_s	w_f
Value in mm	12.5	14.5	4	12	10.2	0.45

Parameters	l_f	w_1	w_2	w_3	l_d	l_e
Value in mm	4.325	0.5	1.17	0.65	1	9.5

Though a compact size of the M3-1 antenna has been achieved, an even smaller antenna size is of significance for the IMDs. Based on this model, two further miniaturization techniques are introduced in the following sections. It has already been discussed that the coupling between the meandered strips and the ground is essential for the radiation of the E-fields. To optimize this coupling, the slot in section 4.2.2 and the meandered strips in section 4.2.3 are modified. The goal is to lower the resonance frequency by optimizing the electrical coupling between meandered strips and slot. In this way, a small-sized antenna can be achieved, while maintaining the resonance frequency.

4.2.2. Stripline-fed slot antenna with modified slotted ground (M3-2)

To miniaturize the antenna M3-1, the circumference of the slotted ground is increased by introducing two strips on the upper edge of both ground layers, which are symmetrical to the center of the antenna structure. In this way, the electrical coupling between the meandered strips and ground is significantly increased, which improves the radiation of the E-fields. In order to maintain a symmetrical radiation characteristic, the dimensions of the strips are selected to be identical and the position must be symmetrical to the center point of the slot.

The new antenna is referred to as the M3-2 antenna and its structure is shown in Figure 4.5. The configuration of Structure 1 and Structure 2 is the same as M3-1 antenna (refer to 4.2 (c)).

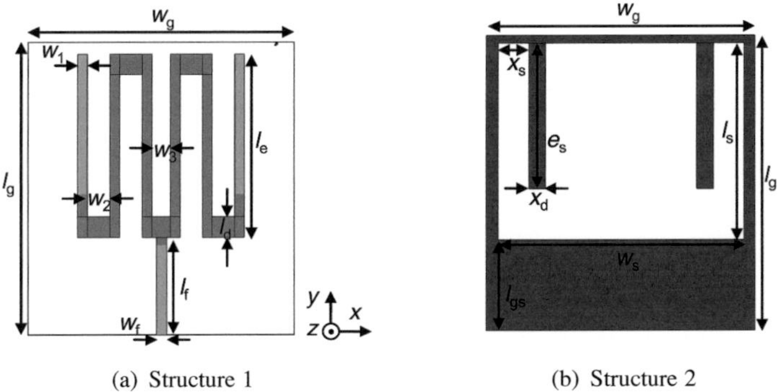

(a) Structure 1   (b) Structure 2

Figure 4.5.: Layout of the antenna M3-2.

To optimize the additionally introduced strips, the influences of the parameters (e_s and x_s) in terms of S_{11} is investigated. The distance x_s is varied in a way that the strips are approximately above the middle of one meandered segment, i.e. at x_s =3.8 mm, the strip is located above the first short upper meandered strip, continuing with x_s =2.7 mm, where the strip is above the second long meandered strip. The results in Figure 4.6 show a decrease of the resonance frequency with a smaller x_s. Furthermore, regarding the impact of the additional metal structures on the radiation pattern, the radiation maximum is split in two maximums in the xz-plane in the case of a large x_s =3.8 mm in simulation (see in Figure 4.7). It is because the intensity of the surface current in the center of the meandered structure decreases. With decreasing x_s, however, the surface current on the inner two meandered arms and on the ground layer (see in Figure 4.8) increases, thus forcing the peaks to converge.

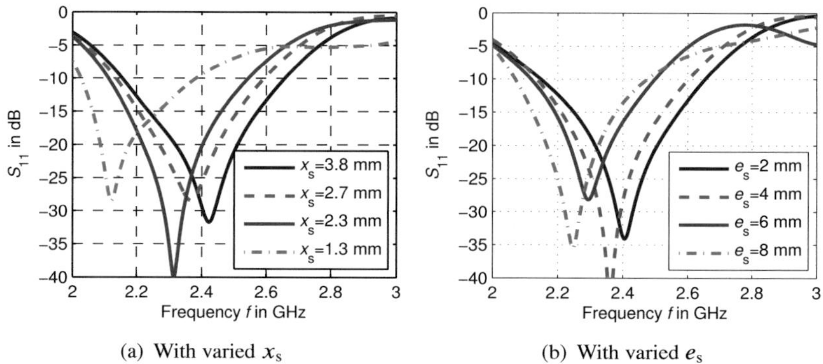

(a) With varied x_s

(b) With varied e_s

Figure 4.6.: Simulated S_{11} of antenna M3-2 with varied x_s and e_s.

Increasing another important parameter, e_s, the resonance frequency decreases (see in Figure 4.6 (b)). However, the larger the e_s, the more skewed the main beam direction from the normal radiation direction towards x direction [You12].

The fully optimized parameters are given in Table 4.4. The antenna has a size of 12.94×11.66 mm^2. In comparison to the formerly proposed M3 antenna, a size reduction of 17.7 % has been achieved.

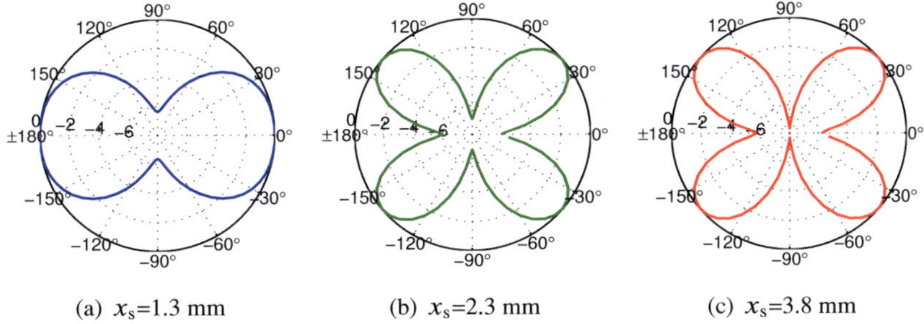

(a) x_s=1.3 mm   (b) x_s=2.3 mm   (c) x_s=3.8 mm

Figure 4.7.: Simulated radiation pattern of antenna M3-2 with varied x_s in yz-plane (normalized in dB).

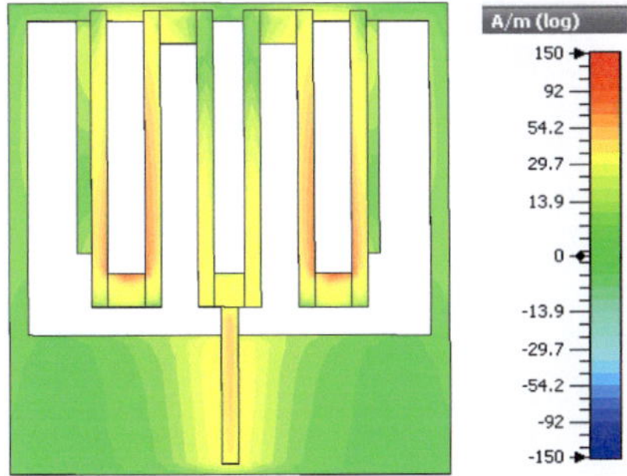

Figure 4.8.: Surface current distribution of the antenna M3-2 (meandered strip with one ground on the bottom side visible): $x_\mathrm{s} = 1.3$ mm and $e_\mathrm{s} = 6$ mm.

Table 4.4.: Parameters of the antenna M3-2.

Parameters	w_g	l_g	w_s	l_s	w_1	w_2	w_3	l_gs
Values in mm	11.66	12.94	10.68	8.62	0.43	0.98	0.82	3.82

Parameters	w_f	l_f	l_d	l_e	x_s	e_s	x_d	-
Values in mm	0.45	4.30	0.91	8.13	1.33	6.38	0.73	-

4.2.3. Stripline-fed slot antenna with modified meandered strips (M3-3)

By applying the second miniaturization technique, the third antenna model (M3-3) is developed. Here, the meandered strips were folded to extend the electrical length of the meandered strips without enlarging its size and to improve the coupling between meandered strips and slotted ground.

The influence of the additional meandered strips on the S_{11}-parameters are shown in Figure 4.10. It is obvious that the enlarged electrical length of the meandered strips is responsible for the decrease of the resonance frequency. The parameter w_4 contributes to the impedance matching and the resonance frequency. A strong decrease of the resonance frequency is observed with the increase of w_4, while the impedance matching is degraded. However, modifying the width w_5, its impact on impedance matching and bandwidth is not significant.

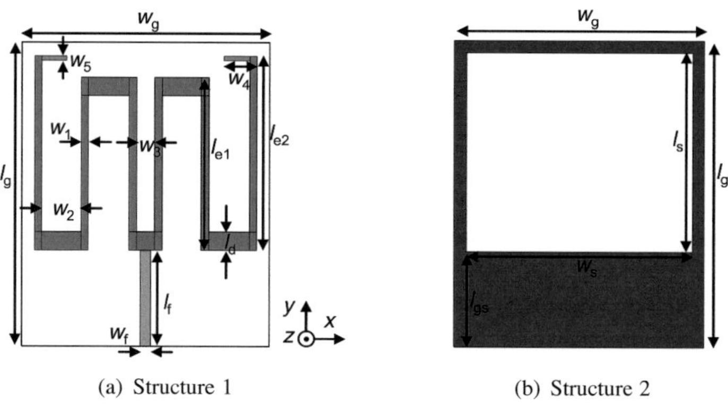

(a) Structure 1   (b) Structure 2

Figure 4.9.: Geometry of the M3-3 antenna.

As can be seen from the parameters in Table 4.5, the optimized M3-3 antenna has an overall size of $12.9 \times 10.15\,\mathrm{mm}^2$, i.e. a size reduction of 27.8 % has been achieved compared to the M3-1 antenna.

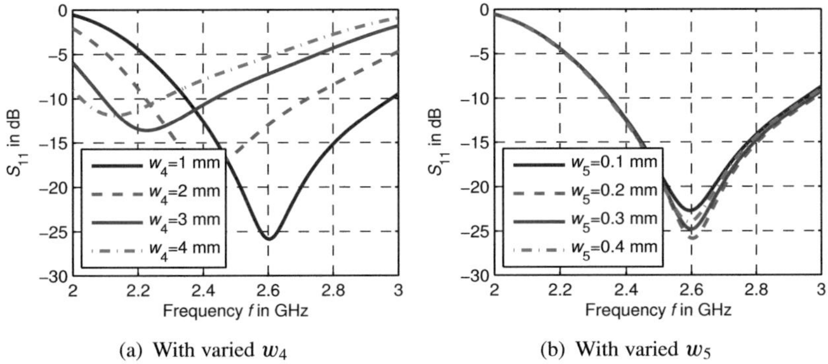

(a) With varied w_4 (b) With varied w_5

Figure 4.10.: Simulated S_{11} of antenna M3-3 with varied w_4 and w_5.

Table 4.5.: Parameters of the antenna M3-3.

Parameters	w_g	l_g	w_s	l_s	w_1	w_2	w_3	l_{gs}
Value in mm	10.15	12.9	9.45	8.4	0.32	1.68	0.77	3.82

Parameters	w_f	l_f	l_d	l_{e1}	l_{e2}	w_4	w_5	-
Value in mm	0.45	4.06	0.79	7.35	8.27	1.37	0.21	-

4.3. Verification of the stripline-fed double-layer slot antennas

In this section, the characteristics of the three stripline-fed double-layer slot antennas will be verified by measurements. For the verification purpose, a solution of water and sugar is chosen to emulate the muscle tissue. The sugar-water solution is very suitable to emulate the muscle tissues (high relative permittivity) within a narrow bandwidth. This is because water and sugar have a dielectric constant of ε_r of 77.2 and 3 at 2.45 GHz [TRVdVG95], respectively. The relative permittivity and conductivity of the muscle tissues can be exactly obtained by mixing sugar and water with a certain weigh ratio. However, the sugar-water mixture cannot emulate each tissue with arbitrary ratio. To emulate tissues with low relative permittivity (e.g. bone), a high weight ratio (> 1:1) of sugar is required, which is not completely soluble in water at room temperature.

To approximate the dielectric property of muscle tissues at 2.45 GHz, the sugar content is finally experimentally determined (40.9%). Table 4.6 depicts the weight ratio of the sugar-water solution for the tissue-equivalent phantom. As can be seen in Figure 4.11, the approximation of the sugar-water solution to muscle is sufficiently precise [GGC96, GLG96a]. Furthermore, an attenuation constant of 4.89 dB/cm at 2.45 GHz can be determined.

Table 4.6.: Recipe for the sugar-water solution to emulate muscle tissues.

Ingredient	weight ratio in %
Water	59.1
Sugar	40.9

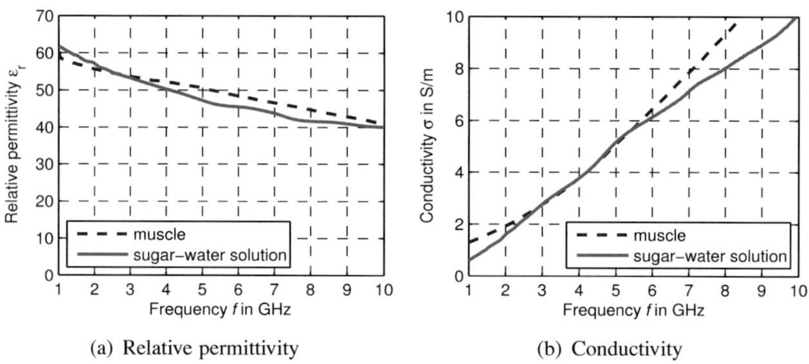

(a) Relative permittivity

(b) Conductivity

Figure 4.11.: Dielectric properties of the sugar-water solution vs. muscle tissue.

The antennas have been fabricated by etching the two substrates separately and then bonding them with glue. To minimize the influence caused by the additional dielectric (glue) between the substrates, the effect of the glue is also examined in the simulation. Figure 4.12 shows the simulation results of the M3-1 antenna in the case of a 0.2 mm thick adhesive layer placed between the two substrates. The conductivity of the muscle tissues is taken into account in the simulation. The blue curve illustrates the S_{11} of the antenna with a homogeneous distribution of the glue between the two substrates. Distributing the glue only along the borderline of the substrate with a width of 2 mm, the S_{11} (red color) is strongly degraded due to the presence of the air gap between two substrates. The green curve shows S_{11} of the antenna, while the glue is distributed only near the boundary of the rectangular substrate. In this case, its influence on S_{11} is very slight. Thus, the last method is chosen for gluing the substrates together.

The antennas are fed by a semi-rigid coaxial cable, which has an inner diameter of 0.9 mm and an outer diameter of 3.58 mm, respectively. Figure 4.13 shows the prototypes of stripline-fed slot antennas. The size reduction of the M3-2 and M3-3 can be clearly seen from the photos. In Figure 4.13 (a), the substrates in the upper row have the Structure 1 (refer to Figure 4.2) on one side and are free of copper on the other side, while the substrates in the lower row are soldered with both Structure 1 and Structure 2. The fabricated prototypes with semi-rigid cables are shown in Figure 4.13 (b). The antennas are immersed in the sugar-water solution to measure the impedance matching of the antennas.

Figure 4.14 provides the measured S_{11} compared with the simulated results. The measured S_{11} of the three antennas agrees very well with the simulated results. The resonance frequency of the measured S_{11} of the M3-1 antenna is the same as the simulated one. However, a strong shift of the resonance frequency of the measured S_{11} of the M3-2 antenna is identified. The S_{11} in the whole ISM band from 2.4 to 2.5 GHz is not sufficiently good (under -10 dB), though the simulated antenna is matched in this frequency range. After fabricating four prototypes, M3-2 indicates very high sensitivity of the performance to the manufacturing tolerance. This is due to the displacement of the two strips placed on the upper edge of both ground layers, which influences the S_{11} and the radiation pattern. Moreover, the shift of the resonance frequency of the antenna M3-3 is acceptable, since the antenna is still matched from 2.4 to 2.5 GHz.

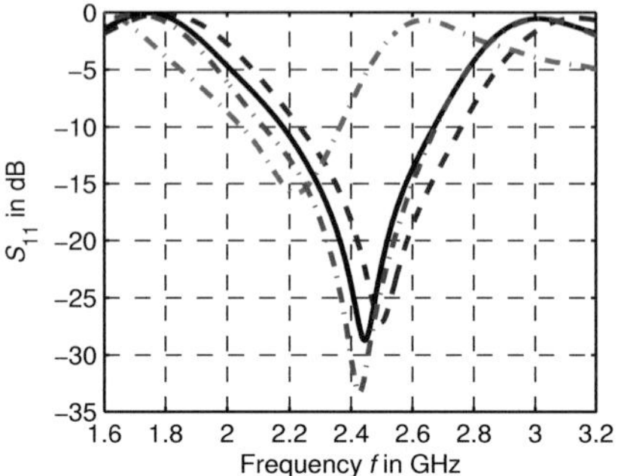

Figure 4.12.: Simulated S_{11} of the antenna M3-1 with different glue distributions between substrates: homogeneous distribution between the substrates (blue), along the borderline of the substrates with a width of 2 mm (red), near the boundary of the substrate (green) and without glue (black).

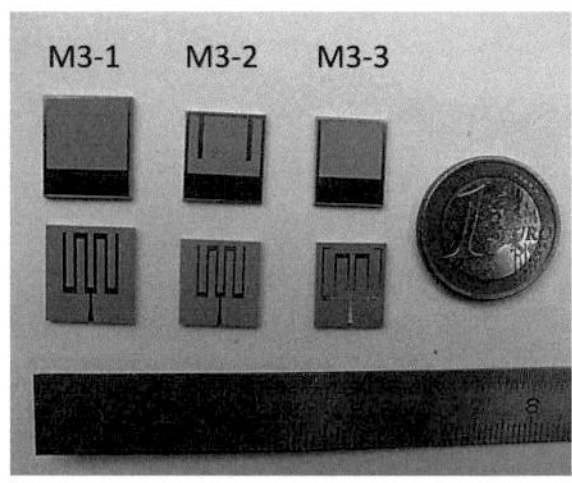

(a) Etched substrates

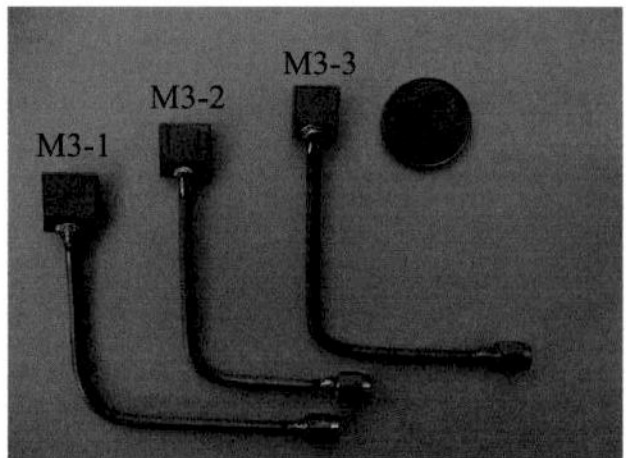

(b) Fabricated antenna prototypes

Figure 4.13.: Photos of the prototypes of the stripline-fed slot antennas.

In the next step, the radiation patterns of the antennas are investigated. It is assumed that the distance between the implantable antenna and the external receiver is more than 50 mm. The radiation pattern of the antennas are characterized at a distance of 70 mm (due to the geometrical limitation for the 360° rotation), which corresponds to the far-field of the antennas (R_{ff}= 18 mm). The experimental setup for antenna pattern measurements is illustrated in Figure 4.15. For the measurements, the coaxial cable is bent (see Figure 4.13) to

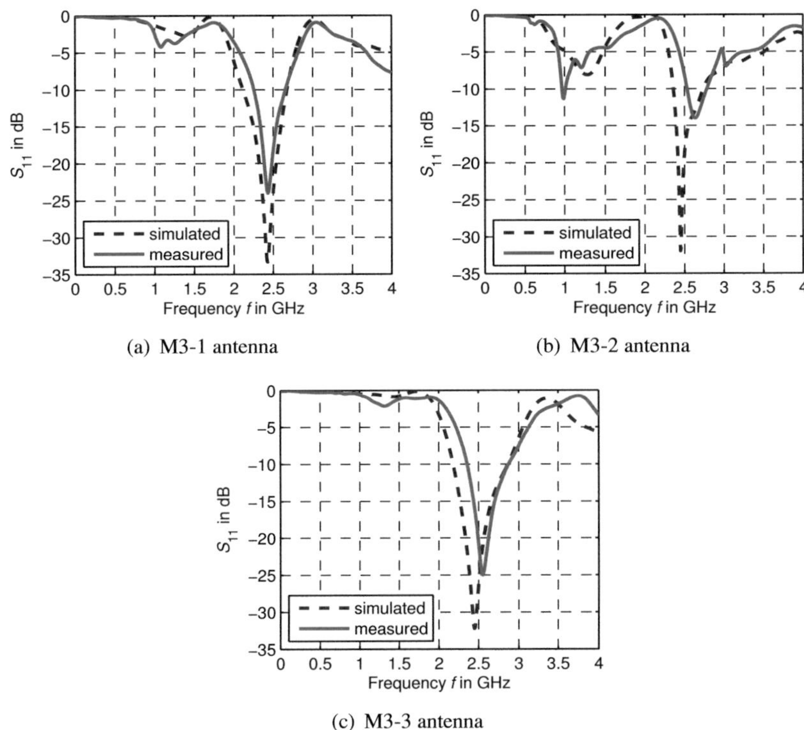

Figure 4.14.: Simulated and measured S_{11} of the three stripline-fed slot antennas.

position the antenna on the platform with motors. The antennas are suspended vertically into sugar-water solution. The used cables are wrapped with tape and polythene foil to waterproof them. The dimensions of the sugar-water container are $40{\times}60{\times}10\,\mathrm{cm}^3$. Based on the respective antenna configurations (see Figure 4.2, 4.5 and 4.9), the E-plane corresponds to the yz-plane, whereas the H-plane is located in the xz-plane.

It can be observed in the measurement that the measured results are strongly influenced by the accuracy of the location of the probe and AUT. The mis-

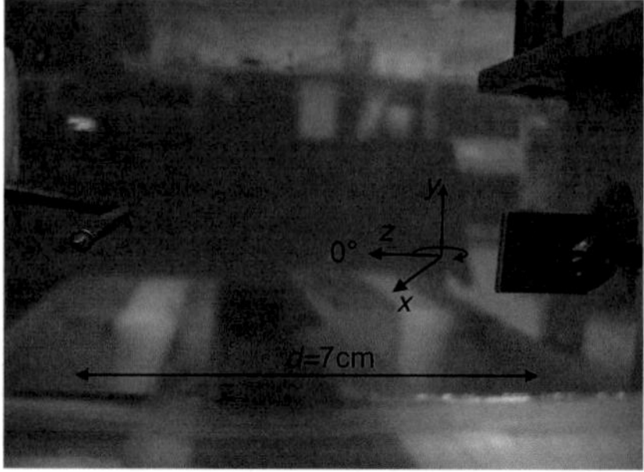

(a) Antenna alignment for E-plane

Figure 4.15.: Measurment setup of radiation pattern for implantable antennas

alignment of the probe and AUT can result in a shift of phase and amplitude, thus further distorting the radiation pattern.

The measured radiation patterns in the E-plane and H-plane of three antennas are shown in Figure 4.16, for co- and cross-polarization. It can be seen that the main beam of the radiation pattern is normal to the surface of the antenna structure (in $\pm z$ directions).

A directive pattern of three antennas in the E-plane is observed. The radiation at 0° and 180° ($\pm x$ axis) is very low. No sidelobes exist in the E-plane. The radiation pattern of the antenna M3-2 is not exactly symmetric. A difference of 8 dB between the two main beam directions at 90° and -90° can be seen. Moreover, in the E-plane, a cross-polarization suppression of more than 20 dB in main beam direction of antenna M3-1 and M3-3 is achieved.

In the H-plane, omni-directional patterns of all the three antennas can be identified. A cross-polarization suppression of 10 dB can be estimated. Different main lobes at multiples of 45° can be observed in cross-polarization. This is because of the surface current existing at the corners of the slotted ground, which causes radiation in cross-polarization in H-plane (xz-plane).

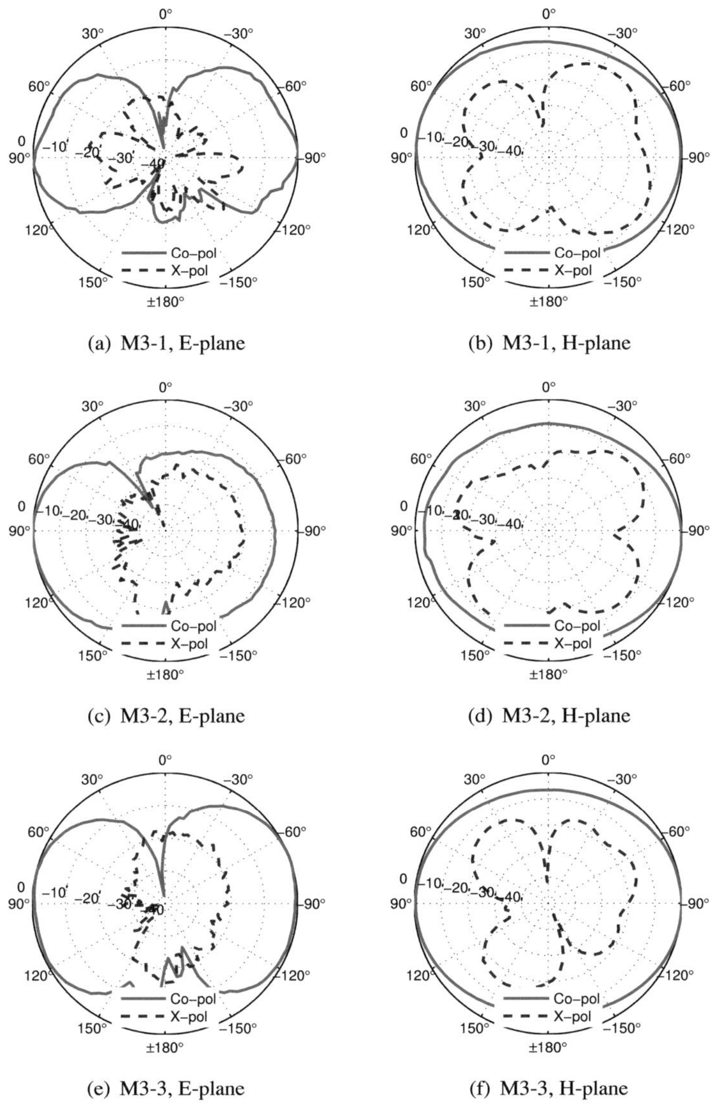

Figure 4.16.: Measured radiation pattern of the implantable antennas at a distance of 70 mm in the E-plane and H-plane at 2.45 GHz (normalized in dB).

4.4. Summary

The design concept of the M3-1 antenna relies on a stripline-feed, meandered strips and a slotted ground to achieve high radiation efficiency, large bandwidth (more than 10%). The radiation efficiency of the antenna is increased by using a stripline-feed, since no surface- and fringing waves are present along the stripline surrounded by a lossy medium and hence additional loss along the feed line is prevented. The meandered strips contribute to the reduction of the antenna size, while the slotted ground improves the antenna bandwidth.

Based on this antenna, the miniaturization of the antenna size to achieve the same resonance frequency was demonstrated by the optimization of the antenna structures. It has been shown that by introducing strips on the ground planes (M3-2 antenna) or extending the meandered strips (M3-3 antenna), the stripline-fed slot antenna can be further miniaturized compared to the size of the M3-1 antenna. The size of the M3-2 antenna was reduced at the expense of a reduced bandwidth and radiation efficiency. The M3-3 antenna with the modified meandered strips is successfully optimized. By the optimization of the antenna structures with regard to the coupling effect and the careful regulation of the current distribution, the antenna size of M3-3 is strongly decreased, while the bandwidth and high radiation efficiency of the antenna are still maintained.

A short overview of the three implantable antennas is given in Table 4.7 with respect to bandwidth (BW), relative bandwidth (rel. BW), peak gain (G_p) ($\sigma = 0\,\mathrm{S/m}$), radiation efficiency (η) in simulations and measurements. Additionally, for comparison, characteristics of two planar implantable antennas optimized for ISM band in [AKS13] and [SKR$^+$11] are given. It can be seen that the antenna M3-3 features the smallest dimensions and the largest bandwidth in both simulation and measurement. The antenna M3-2 has the highest gain in the simulation, however, has the narrowest bandwidth and lowest radiation efficiency with respect to the simulation results. In conclusion, the M3-3 antenna shows the best radiation properties.

The M3-1 and M3-3 antennas fulfilled the requirements mentioned at the beginning of this chapter for IMDs operated at the ISM band. The performance

Table 4.7.: Comparison of the M3-1, M3-2, M3-3, reference antenna 1 in [AKS13] and reference antenna 2 in [SKR$^+$11].

Antenna	M3-1	M3-2	M3-3	ref. 1	ref. 2
Size (mm^2)	14.5×12.5	12.9×11.6	12.9×10.1	11×11	24.6×25.9
Simulated BW (GHz)	2.16-2.68 = 0.52	2.36-2.74 = 0.37	2.27-2.89 = 0.625	2.34-2.52 = 0.18	2.30-2.57 = 0.27
Rel. BW	19.5%	17.7%	32.15%	7.4%	11%
Simulated η	98.9%	84.6%	94.2%	-	-
Measured BW (GHz)	2.25-2.6 = 0.35	2.53-2.78 = 0.25	2.36-2.87 = 0.51	- -	2.20-2.55 = 0.35
Rel. BW	14.4%	9.4%	19.5%	-	14.2%

of these implantable antennas is successfully verified by measurements. The characterized radiation patterns are omni-directional in the H-plane and directional in the E-plane with high directivity, which enables the establishment of a robust wireless link between the IMDs and external medical devices. Moreover, the developed implantable antennas with compact size will lead to small-sized IMDs, which will significantly improve the applicability of IMDs.

This closes the chapter on the design of the implantable antennas for wireless communication of IMDs. Regarding the second medical application (i.e. medical diagnosis), the design details of the on-body matched antennas can be found in the next chapter.

5. On-body matched antennas for medical diagnosis

In this chapter, we move on from the implantable antennas to on-body matched antennas. These on-body matched antennas address the drawbacks of off-body antennas (as discussed in chapter 2) for microwave medical diagnosis purposes. In contrast with implantable antennas discussed in the previous chapter, the antennas for medical diagnosis are required to feature a very wide bandwidth to allow a high-resolution imaging based on radar imaging. In microwave tomography, traditionally mono-frequency procedure is applied and narrow band antennas can be used. However, a multifrequency (or wideband) processing improves the inversion results hence the imaging quality [GMZ$^+$10]. Therefore, the goal of this chapter is to develop wideband and multi-band antennas.

Different on-body matched antennas operating in two different frequency ranges for medical diagnosis are presented. First, the challenges and design principles of the on-body matched antennas are described. In the following sections, different differentially-fed wideband slot antennas with different slot-shapes for the miniaturization of the antenna size are discussed and compared. These antennas are characterized from 1 to 7 GHz. To enhance the sensitivity of the system with respect to weak reflections from targets in human tissues, a lower operational frequency is required. Therefore, a dual-band slotted Bowie antenna (characterized from 0.5 to 0.7 GHz and 1.3 to 4 GHz) and a folded Bowtie antenna (characterized from 0.5 to 2 GHz) are designed with the focus on miniaturization and stable radiation properties.

5.1. Motivation and design challenges of on-body matched antennas

Microwave medical diagnosis via imaging for the identification of e.g. tumors is based on the concept of observing the reflected signal from the target (in some methods, the transmission is also utilized). The reflections are caused by the contrast of the dielectric properties between the tumor and the surrounding healthy tissues. For the detection of these reflections, high radiation penetration of the signals from the antenna into the human body is desirable to achieve a high SNR, since the reflections are very weak due to the high signal attenuation in tissues (see chapter 2). For such applications, the performance of the antennas is the governing factor of the overall system performance. Matching the antennas on the human body has the purpose of reducing the strong reflection from the air-skin interface (drawback of the off-body antennas discussed in chapter 1) and to allow more energy to penetrate into the human body to obtain a stronger signal for image processing. Another advantage of matching the antenna to the human body is that the size can be rescaled according to the relative permittivity of the human skin, since the high relative permittivity leads to a wavelength shorter than in free space. However, the antenna design for medical diagnosis differs from that for regular antennas for free-space operation due to the presence of the complex human body, which can be modeled as a lossy medium. Therefore several challenges arise in the design stage. The general design challenges of body-matched antennas have been mentioned in the introduction. In detail, the following challenges and requirements are associated with the design of on-body matched wideband antennas for medical diagnosis:

- **Operational frequency** The operational frequency of the antenna should preferably include low frequencies (around 1 GHz) considering the high-contrast characteristic and low signal attenuation in human tissues.

- **Operational bandwidth** The operational bandwidth must be as large as possible to achieve a high range resolution, since the range resolution is inversely proportional to the operational bandwidth. That means the larger the bandwidth, the finer the range resolution.

- **Radiation property** The radiation property must not change significantly in the whole frequency band. The near-field pattern must be investigated. A high radiation efficiency of the antennas is desirable.

- **Front-to-back ratio** A high front-to-back ratio of the antenna radiation and low side- and back-radiation are desired to minimize the antenna coupling and the interference to other microwave sub-systems. This also allows a high portion of energy to be coupled into the human body.

- **Reflection between air and human skin** Since the antenna should be optimized for operation directly on the skin, a good contact between the antenna and skin is needed. The sensitivity of the antenna performance regarding imperfect contact must be investigated. In the case of a non-flat surface such as the skin on head with hairs, matching materials should be used.

- **Antenna size** For medical diagnosis, an antenna array with a number of antenna elements both for transmitting and receiving is typically applied. The small-sized antenna allows the construction of an array with a large number of elements within limited area/space for gathering more useful reflections. In this way, a microwave image with high quality (e.g. signal-to-clutter ratio (SCR)) can be obtained. More details will be discussed in chapter 6.

- **Verification by measurement** The variation of the permittivity of tissues results in a significant change of performance of the antenna. Hence a similar scenario and boundary conditions in the simulation and measurement are required. The antenna must be water-tight for the measurement of the radiation pattern. The measurements of antennas (i.e. S_{11}) are performed in tissue-simulating liquid as well as on the human skin.

5.2. Design procedure

Since the on-body matched antennas are in direct contact with the human body, the behavior of the antennas depends on the dielectric properties and geometry of the human body. Therefore, the antennas should be optimized together with the human body model in the design procedure. However, a simulation of antennas with the human body model results in high number of mesh cells and a simulation time of a few days is expected. Due to the limitation of the memory capacity and computational capability of the computer, it is not recommended to optimize the antenna together with a whole complex human model with a high space resolution. The duration of antenna optimization will be extremely long. Therefore, an efficient optimization procedure for the on-body matched antennas is required.

The optimization procedure of the antenna in the configuration shown in Figure 5.1 is performed in CST Microwave studio with the following steps:

- Step 1: The antenna is constructed together with a free space region on one side. On the other side of the antenna is a tissue-simulating phantom as shown in Figure 5.1 (a). The phantom has the averaged relative permittivity of skin and fat [GLG96a]. The frequency dispersion and conductivity of the phantom material (ε_r= 20 or 35 depending on the frequency bands, σ=0 S/m) is not considered. The open boundary condition is used in the simulation so that the reflection on the boundary is ignored. Therefore, the impedance matching, efficiency and gain of the antenna can be investigated. Since many iterations are required, the considerations above can significantly reduce the number of mesh cells thus reducing the computing time per iteration.

- Step 2: The antenna is simulated with the free space region on one side and a realistic tissue-simulating phantom including its frequency dispersion and conductivity. A parameter tuning is performed with the experience from the parameter study in step 1. The impedance matching and radiation pattern of the antenna are investigated. The parameters of the antenna are then updated.

- Step 3: A further study (i.e. SAR) of the antenna together with a complicated multilayer human phantom shown in Figure 5.1 (b) is performed. In this configuration, the realistic permittivities of different tissues and the multi-reflections of different layers are taken into account.

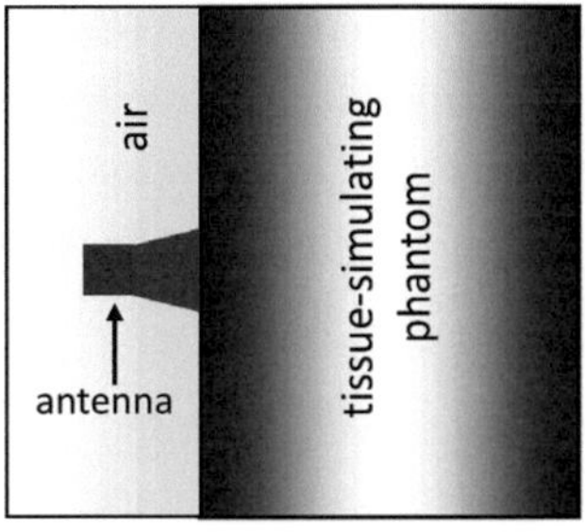

(a) With tissue-simulating phantom

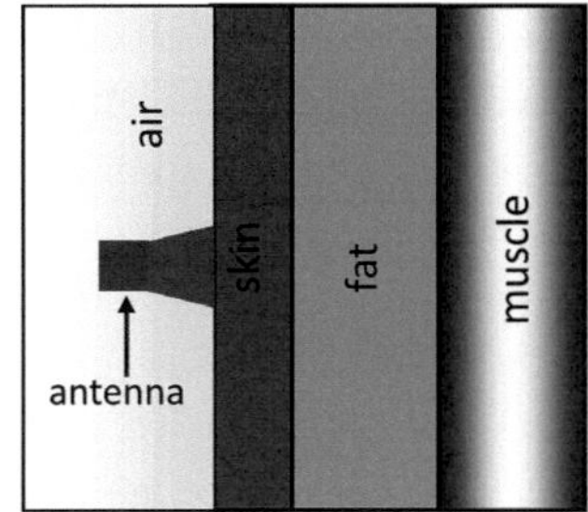

(b) With multilayer human phantom

Figure 5.1.: Simulation scenarios of the on-body matched antenna with tissue-simulating phantom and multilayer human phantom.

The final optimized parameters can be imported into the models in step 1 and 2 to obtain different characteristics of the antenna (gain, radiation pattern, etc.). After the optimization steps, the antennas are fabricated for the verification by measurement with respect to the impedance matching and radiation pattern in the tissue-simulating liquid. The tissue-simulating liquid emulates the dielectric properties of the human tissues. A slight modification of the antenna dimensions can be made after the analysis of the measured results.

After introducing of the challenges and the design principle of the on-body matched wideband antennas, different concepts of developing these antennas are described in the following sections. The antennas are characterized in different operational frequency bands with the focus on the miniaturization of the antennas.

5.3. Differentially-fed slot antennas for the operational band from 1 to 7 GHz

Taking the challenges and requirements in section 5.1 into account, a planar antenna structure is applied for the easy and low-cost fabrication of the antennas. Moreover, the planar antenna can be also easily contacted to the nearly planar surface of human body. Regarding the radiation pattern, most on-body antennas suffer from the problem of the beam width and main beam direction varying over frequency as well as over the changing permittivity of the human tissues. To achieve a stable main beam direction in the whole frequency range, symmetrical radiating element with differential feed is adopted. The goal is to obtain a sufficiently large bandwidth and high radiation efficiency as well as a good penetration into human tissues.

In this section, the design of UWB slot antennas based on the concept in [ABWZ09, Ada10] using a new design procedure and miniaturization technique, is investigated. The antenna is characterized from 1 to 7 GHz (lower frequencies refer from 1 to 3 GHz, while higher frequencies are from 3 GHz in the later discussion). Due to the large wavelength at 1 GHz, three different slots for the miniaturization of the antenna size are investigated and verified both in simulation and measurement: double elliptical slot, sector-like slot and stepped slot, which are discussed in succession in the following sections. Then, an optimized feed network is introduced to reduce the overall size of the antennas.

5.3.1. Double-elliptical slot antenna

To maintain a symmetrical structure, two elliptically shaped monopoles on the top and a double-elliptical slotted ground at the bottom of the antenna are designed. The double-elliptical shape is used to miniaturize the antenna.

In Figure 5.2, the layout of the double-elliptical slot antenna fed by microstrip lines is shown. The antenna consists of two elliptically shaped monopoles on the top side of the substrate surrounded by a double-elliptically slotted ground plane (the inverse area of the double elliptical slot) at the bottom side. In the preliminary design, the elliptically shaped monopoles are differentially fed by two tapered microstrip lines with $50\,\Omega$ line impedance at the ports. The input signals at the two ports have a $180°$ phase difference. Therefore, the radiated co-polarized E-fields related to both monopoles are in phase [31]. Instead of the differential feed with microstrip lines, a differentially-fed network (refer to Figure 5.4) used to feed the two monopoles will be introduced later.

The symmetrical arrangement of the two monopoles each within one slot helps to keep the current distribution in the radiation zone symmetrical around the center of the antenna. Such a current distribution results in a symmetri-

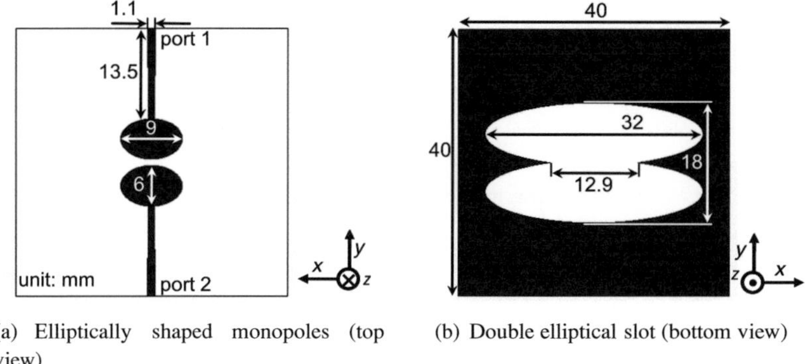

(a) Elliptically shaped monopoles (top view)

(b) Double elliptical slot (bottom view)

Figure 5.2.: The layout of the double-elleptical slot antenna.

cal radiation pattern, which can be optimized to be very stable over the operational frequency range. In this way the phase center (whose position is frequency independent) of the radiation is located exactly in between the two monopoles at the center of the structure due to the symmetry of the current distribution [ABWZ09]. This indicates that the radiating impulse of this antenna features a low distortion and a high fidelity.

The lowest operational frequency of the slotted wideband antenna can generally be written as

$$f_\mathrm{L} = \frac{c_0}{C_\mathrm{s}\sqrt{\varepsilon_\mathrm{r,eff}}} \tag{5.1}$$

where C_s is the circumference of the slot and $\varepsilon_\mathrm{r,eff}$ is the effective relative permittivity of the substrate. Therefore, to achieve a low operation frequency, either a large circumference of the slot or a high-permittivity substrate should be used.

Compared to a single elliptical slot with the same dimensions, the double-elliptical slot on the ground plane with the same length and width increases the circumference, thus lowering the operation frequency without changing the overall size of the antenna. As a result, the lower operational frequency is further decreased and the overall bandwidth is increased.

On the other hand, a high-permittivity substrate is desirable for the miniaturization of the antenna. However, the relative permittivity of the commercially available low-profile substrates is limited up to around 10 due to the high fabrication cost. To increase the relative permittivity of the substrate (larger than 15), ceramic body combining using sintering technology is proposed in [dCHS$^+$11]. The size of the antenna can be rescaled due to the high relative permittivity and therefore be miniaturized. In this work, the substrate Rogers RT 6010 (PTFE/Ceramic Laminates) with the dielectric constant of 10.2 and thickness of 1.27 mm is chosen for the antenna design and the fabrication. This substrate does not feature an extremely high relative permittivity compared to ceramic substrates. However, the antenna structure can easily be etched. The miniaturization of the antenna is based on the optimization of the antenna structure including the feed network with regard to the current distribution of the antenna.

Since the antenna is matched to the human body, the high relative permittivity of the tissues contribute to the high effective permittivity $\varepsilon_{r,eff}$ of the antenna. In simulation, a phantom emulating the human body is placed on the ground side as in Figure 5.3 (a), leaving free space on the top side of the substrate. The phantom ($\varepsilon_r = 20$, $\sigma = 0$ S/m) has the average relative permittivity of skin and fat at 4 GHz (center frequency of the operational band from 1 to 7 GHz) [GLG96a] and the dispersion of the phantom material is not considered for the characterization of the antenna. This configuration results in a shorter wavelength within the phantom (as compared to in free space) therefore allowing for a smaller-sized antenna. The direction of the radiation is perpendicular to the ground plane ($+z$ direction) and goes into the phantom. By matching the antenna to the phantom with a high relative permittivity, a directive antenna pattern with high front-to-back ratio can be achieved.

In the optimization procedure, it can be found that the impedance matching at the higher frequencies can be easily achieved. However, an unstable radiation pattern occurs because the wavelength at the higher frequencies is 3 to 4 times smaller than that at the lower frequencies. The current distribution at the higher frequencies changes and a high antenna mode of operation, with side-/grating lobes can be observed. The main pattern in yz-plane is split into different maxima (sidelobes and grating lobes). This can be minimized by reducing the size of the slot and the distance of the two elliptically shaped monopoles in the y direction. Overall, the slot width is increased only in the x direction so that a small distance between two monopoles and the slot edges can be maintained. In this way, the grating lobes are suppressed at the higher frequencies and a desirable radiation pattern can be realized for a wide frequency range.

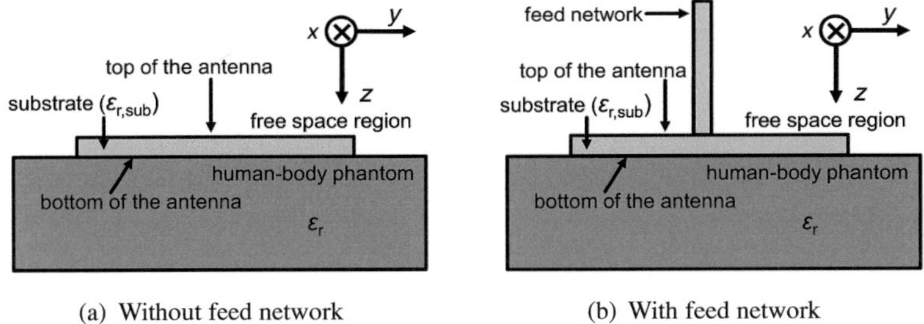

(a) Without feed network

(b) With feed network

Figure 5.3.: The arrangement of the double-elleptical slot antenna and phantom.

In practice, two differential signals must be fed to the two ports of the antenna. Two RF cables for two ports must also be exactly the same to maintain their 180° phase difference. To eliminate this feeding issue, an additional differential feed network is desirable to be connected directly to the antenna element. The differential feed network [ABWZ09] is a wideband divider with differential outputs applied to excite the differential signals. It is made from the same substrate as the antenna to minimize the attenuation caused by the interconnection between the feed network and the antenna. The feed network with a size of $52{\times}26{\times}1.27$ mm^3 is shown in Figure 5.4 (a) and is optimized for the operation from 1 to 10 GHz.

To connect the feed network with the antenna element, the ground plane of the antenna element is moved to the top side as shown in Figure 5.4 (b). The connection of the feed network and the antenna is in such a way that the ports 2 and 3 in Figure 5.4 (a) are connected to the respective port of the same label in Figure 5.4 (b). For the differential feed setup, the microstrip line at port 2 is connected to the monopole while the ground of port 3 is connected to the

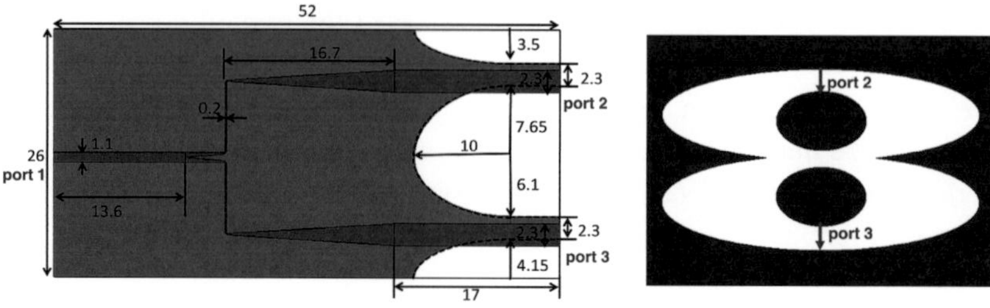

(a) Feed network (top and bottom sides superimposed) (b) Radiator element on top side

Figure 5.4.: The layout of the double elliptical slot antenna and differential feed network (condcutors are grey; unit: mm).

monopole. The feed signal is channeled into the feed network from port 1. Figure 5.5 illustrates the perspective view of the slot antenna together with the feed network.

The arrangement of the antenna element and feed network is illustrated in Figure 5.3 (b). With this configuration, the signals are radiated perpendicularly to the surface of the underside of the antenna (without the ground plane) into human body. The overall size of the antenna is $26{\times}35{\times}52\,\mathrm{mm}^3$.

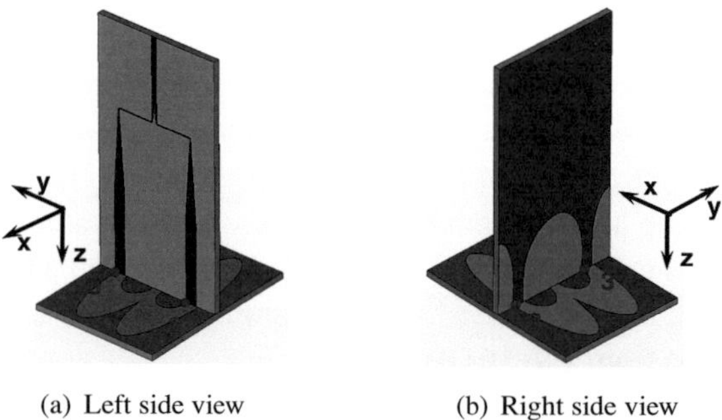

(a) Left side view (b) Right side view

Figure 5.5.: The perspective view of double-elliptical slot antenna with feed network (circular points indicate the electrical connections between feed network and radiating element).

Characteristics of the double-elliptical slot antenna

In the following section, the characteristics of the optimized antenna model in simulation will be given to demonstrate the achievements of the discussed design principles. The simulation results will be then verified by measurement.

The simulated input reflection coefficient (S_{11} and S_{22}) at the differential feed ports of the antenna without the feed network (see Figure 5.2) are the same due to the symmetry of the antenna structure. The result (see Figure 5.6 (a)) shows that a very good impedance matching (-10 dB) is achieved in the frequency range from 1.2 to 9 GHz. The curve of S_{11} without strong resonance is observed due to the smooth impedance matching between microstrip feed line and elliptical monopoles.

In Figure 5.6 (b), the impedance matching of the antenna with the feed network (as shown in Figure 5.4) from 1.1 to 9 GHz can be observed. However, the feed network introduces oscillations/resonances due to the feed structure and interconnection with the antenna element. The measurement is performed in the PEG-water solution as mentioned in Chapter 3. A slight difference between the simulated and measured curves, especially around 2 GHz, is observed. It is because the required interpolation of material property in CST leads to slightly different dielectric property of the PEG-water solution compared to the measured one. Moreover, the dispersion of the PEG-water solution at the open boundary in simulation causes also different results. All the body-matched antennas are associated with these two reasons causing slightly different results between simulation and measurement, which will not be repeated in the following chapters. However, the simulated and measured result in PEG-water solution agree well in terms of nulls. At the higher frequencies, the S_{11} is improved to be better than -10 dB. The measured results on the skin and in PEG-water solution are consistent with each other, which shows the applicability of the antenna in direct contact with the skin for medical diagnosis. In the later paragraphs, the differentially-fed slot antennas are referred to the antennas with feed network, if the antennas without feed network are not mentioned.

Since the dielectric properties of human tissues vary across individuals, the sensitivity of the on-body matched antenna to a dielectric property variation is

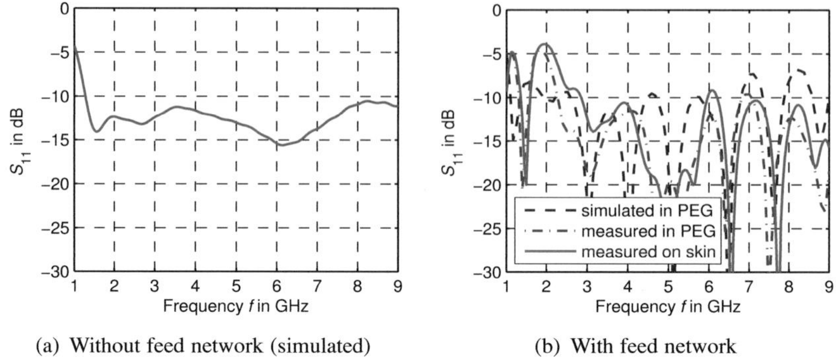

Figure 5.6.: Simulated and measured S_{11} of double-elliptical slot antenna without (fed by microstrip lines) and with feed network.

investigated in the simulation. The variation of relative permittivity of phantom from 20 to 30 are within the normal range of averaged tissue (skin and fat). The results shown in Figure 5.7 confirm that the impedance matching of the proposed antenna is very stable over a large range (from 15 to 30) of relative permittivity of human tissues. This is because the radiating element is located on the top side of the antenna between free space and substrate, hence the change of the relative permittivity of the phantom does not cause a significant variation of the current distribution of the radiating elements especially at the higher frequencies. However, it also can be observed that the S_{11} of the antenna input port at around 2 GHz goes slightly up to -8 dB with high relative permittivity of the phantom.

To investigate the power that penetrates into the phantom (human body), the penetration efficiency η_p is defined as

$$\eta_p = \frac{P_{\text{body}}}{P_{\text{body}} + P_{\text{air}}}, \tag{5.2}$$

where P_{body} and P_{air} are the total radiated power into the human body and in free space region (refer to 5.3 (b)), respectively.

The ratio of the radiation energy into the human body can be also described by the front-to-back ratio. The front-to-back ratio indicates the ratio of radiated

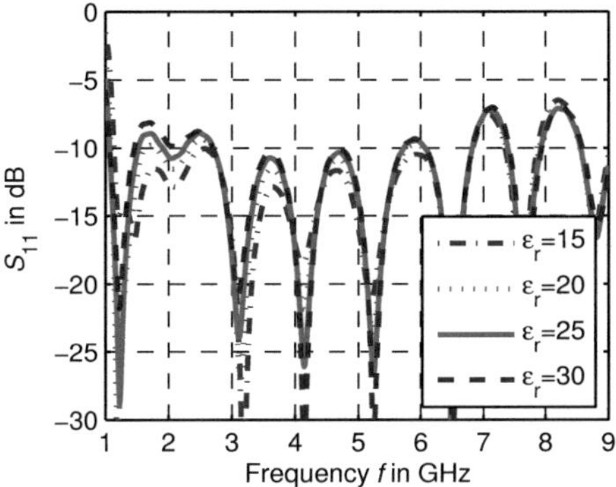

Figure 5.7.: Simulated S_{11} of the double-elliptical slot antenna with varied relative permittivity ε_r of phantom (σ =0 S/m).

power between the front and rear of a directional antenna (the front side of the antenna points to the human body), which is defined as

$$F/B = \frac{P_{\text{body}}}{P_{\text{air}}}. \tag{5.3}$$

It can be seen from (5.3) that a high penetration efficiency yields a high front-to-back ratio.

The penetration efficiency of the double-elliptical slot antenna with varying relative permittivity of the phantom is investigated. The results (see Figure 5.8) show that, in case of $\varepsilon_r = 1$, a penetration efficiency of only about 50% is obtained. Increasing the relative permittivity of the phantom to 10, η_p is mostly above 80%. However, η_p increases slightly with the increasing relative permittivity (from 10 to 40) of the phantom. The reason is, as discussed in the last paragraph, that the radiator is placed between free space region and the substrate with $\varepsilon_{r,\text{sub}} = 10.2$ and thus the dielectric contrast of materials placed on the two sides of radiator cannot be changed significantly by the relative permittivity of phantom. At 7 GHz, the radiation into free space increases at the higher ε_r (e.g. 30). On the other hand, η_p for a relative permittivity of the phantom from 10 to 40 is relatively high (> 0.7) in the whole operating frequency range. It can be concluded that the high η_p is achieved due to the configuration of the antenna in direct contact with the human body. The relative permittivity of tissues (larger than 20) will not affect strongly η_p of the proposed slot antenna.

With $\varepsilon_\mathrm{r} = 20$, 80% of the radiated energy (refer to Figure 5.9) is coupled into the phantom, which indicates a front-to-back ratio of larger than 6 dB. From 3 to 6 GHz, the antenna has a η_p of about 0.9 (F/B >9.5 dB). It can be therefore noted that the double-elliptical slot antenna in direct contact with human body features a high penetration efficiency and front-to-back ratio.

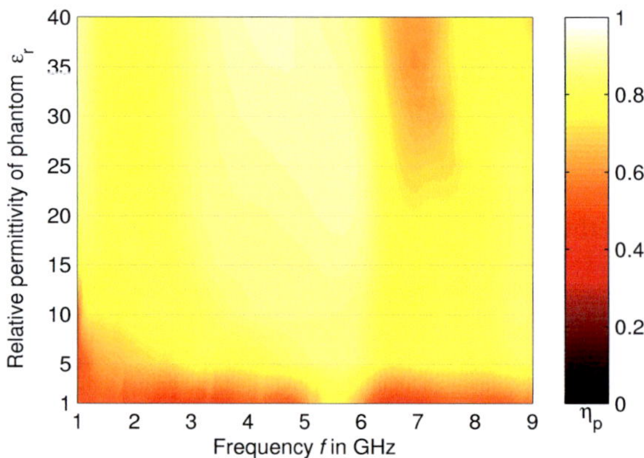

Figure 5.8.: Simulated penetration efficiency η_p (in linear scale) of the double-elliptical slot antenna over frequency with varied relative permittivity ε_r of phantom (σ =0 S/m).

Although the radiation gain (far-field) cannot be achieved in the real scenario due to the presence of lossy human tissues, this is a measure of the designed antenna regarding its radiation efficiency and directivity. The simulated maximum gain of the antenna in the main beam direction with the phantom is shown in Figure 5.9. The results show that the antenna has a relatively high and very constant gain (> 8 dBi) from 2 to 8 GHz. A smaller gain is observed at the lower frequencies. It is due to the antenna being electrically small in terms of wavelength at the lower frequencies, which results in a broad beamwidth of the radiation pattern without a high directivity. On the other hand, the radiation above 7 GHz is not applicable, since the reflection from the targets is too weak to be detected due to the very high signal attenuation. Yet for the operational band from 1 to 7 GHz, the antenna features a very high radiation gain compared to conventional wideband antennas in free space.

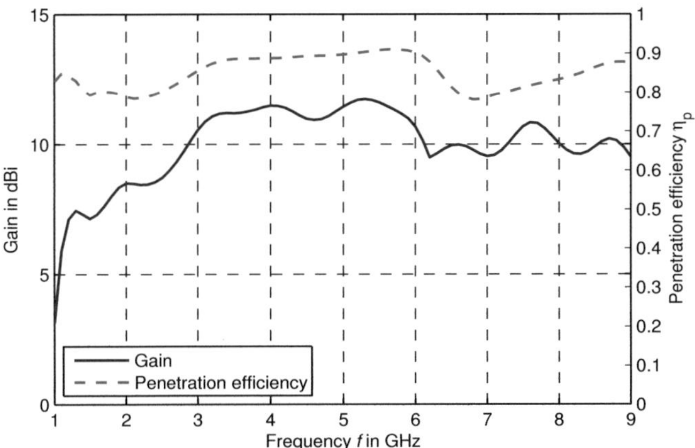

Figure 5.9.: Simulated maximum gain and penetration efficiency of the double-elliptical slot antenna with the phantom ($\varepsilon_r = 20$, $\sigma = 0$ S/m).

Since the antenna is in direct contact with the human body, it is of significance to characterize the near-field pattern. However, the standard free space antenna measurement cannot be used and hence the measurement is performed in the PEG-water solution with a similar dielectric property as the human body. For the measurement, the antenna has to be watertight (shown in Figure 3.8) so that the free space region on the top side will not be affected by the tissue-simulating liquid.

The simulated and measured near-field (R_{ff}=63 mm at 1 GHz, r= 40 mm) pattern in the E-plane and H-plane in PEG-water solution at different frequencies are shown in Figure 5.10 and 5.11, respectively. This distance corresponds to the average thickness of fat and muscle tissues of the human abdomen. The results are limited to 4 GHz due to a high signal attenuation in PEG-water solution at the higher frequencies in the measurement and the VNA used for measurement has a limited dynamic range. From the results, it can be observed that the differential feed and the symmetry of the antenna geometry provide a good symmetrical near-field pattern of the antenna. The radiation direction of the main beam is found to be very stable over a broad frequency range due to the phase center being in the middle of the antenna.

Slight differences (e.g. directivity and side lobes) between simulated and measured results are caused by different boundary condition. To reduce the simulation time, the calculated volume is strongly reduced using open boundary (reflections at the boundary are not considered) in CST compared to the measurement scenario. Moreover, an automatic interpolation of the frequency-dependent permittivity of the medium must be tolerated in the simulation tool to enable the convergence of the solver. However, the similar run of the curves between simulated and measured results is used for the verification purpose.

In the E-plane (yz-plane), a narrow beam is identified with increasing frequency. At 3 GHz and 4 GHz, the pattern features sidelobes as expected in the analysis mentioned in the design principle of this antenna. A wider pattern is observed in the simulation than in the measurement. This is because the measured scenario is not exactly the same as the open boundary in the simulation. It is also due to the high sensitivity of the measured results to the geometrical arrangement of the AUT as mentioned in 3.2.1. In the H-plane (xz-plane), a very similar shape of the near-field patterns can be seen at different frequencies. The beamwidth of the near-field pattern becomes wider with increasing frequency.

It can be concluded that the double-elliptical slot antenna in direct contact with human body exhibits a very good impedance matching from 1.35 to 9 GHz. This antenna features good impedance matching, very high gain, front-to-back ratio and hence very good penetration ability into human body based on the simulation results. Observing the near-field pattern of the antenna, a stable main beam direction is expected due to the symmetric radiating structure. Regarding the simulated gain and pattern, the operational band of the antenna is limited to 7 GHz due to strong sidelobes and grating lobes at the higher frequencies. Based on the analysis in chapter 2, the reflections at the higher frequencies above 7 GHz are too weak to be detected. Hence, the double-elliptical slot antenna with a size of $26 \times 35 \times 52 \, \text{mm}^3$ can be operated

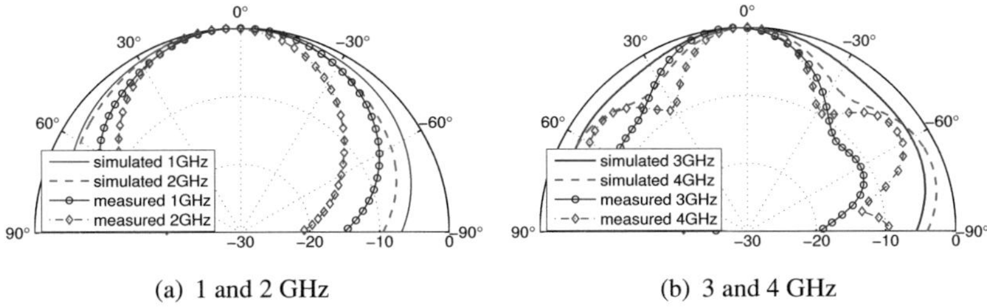

(a) 1 and 2 GHz (b) 3 and 4 GHz

Figure 5.10.: Simulated and measured near-field pattern of the double-elliptical slot antenna (r= 40 mm), E-plane (yz-plane) for co-polarization (normalized in dB).

in frequency range of 1.35 to 7 GHz for medical diagnostic purposes.

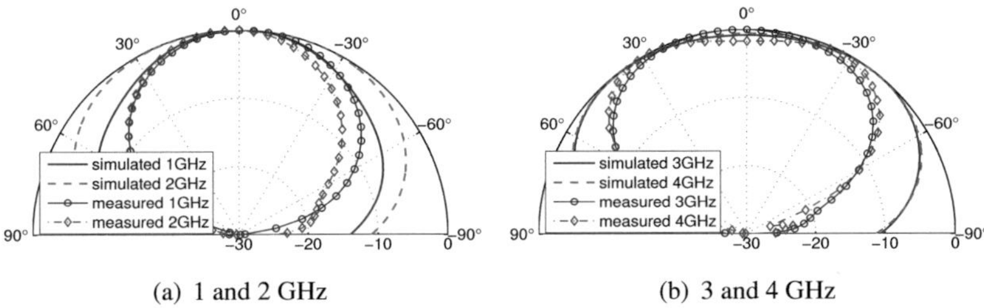

(a) 1 and 2 GHz (b) 3 and 4 GHz

Figure 5.11.: Simulated and measured near-field pattern of the double-elliptical slot antenna (r= 40 mm), H-plane (xz-plane) for co-polarization (normalized in dB).

5.3.2. Sector-like slot antenna

To further increase the circumference of the slot and hence decrease the lowest operational frequency of the antenna from the previous section, the antenna is modified by using a sector-like slot. The sector-like slot antenna is also fabricated on the substrate Rogers RT 6010 (ε_r =10.2 , d =1.27 mm, $\tan \delta$ =0.0023) and has two monopoles and a sector-like slot on the top of the

Table 5.1.: Design parameters of the sector-like slot antenna.

parameter	w	l	s_1	s_2	e_1	e_2	r	α
value (mm)	35	35	1.8	2.2	4.5	3	16	15°

substrate as shown in Figure 5.12 [34].

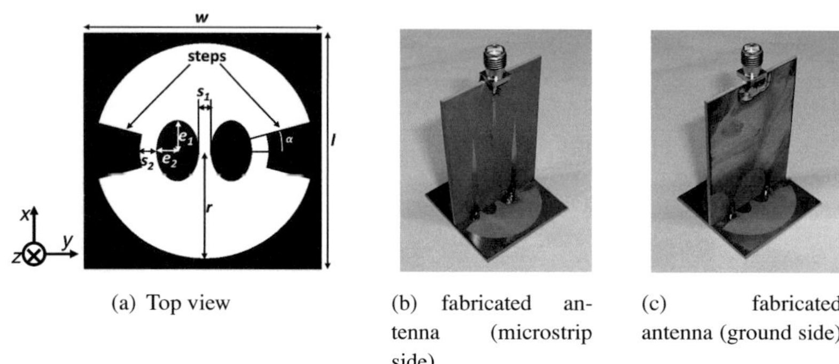

(a) Top view   (b) fabricated antenna (microstrip side)   (c) fabricated antenna (ground side)

Figure 5.12.: Layout and photos of the sector-like slot antenna (conductors are grey).

The parameter s_2 in Figure 5.12 is important for the radiation at high frequencies since a strong surface current at high frequencies is observed at the two steps being closed to the monopoles. The impedance matching of the input port in the whole frequency band is achieved by optimizing e_1, e_2, α, s_1 and s_2. The optimized values of the parameters are given in Table 5.1. The steps between the two sectors are introduced to suppress the high mode current distribution at high frequencies that result in significant sidelobes and grating lobes in the radiation pattern as mentioned in the previous section. By using these steps, the distance between two monopoles s_1 can be reduced (maintain the radius of the slot), which leads to suppress the sidelobes and grating lobes at the higher frequencies [Yan11] [34].

The two monopoles are fed by the same differential feed network from the previous section. The arrangement of the antenna and the feed network is shown in Figure 5.12 (b) and (c). The arrangement of antenna, feed network

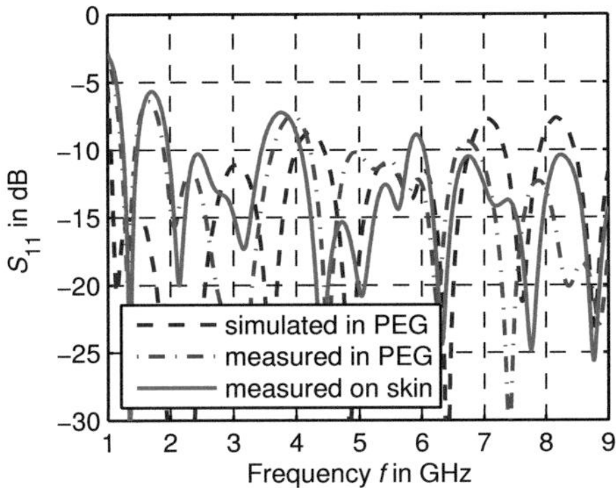

Figure 5.13.: Simulated and measured S_{11} in PEG-water solution of the sector-like slot antenna.

and phantom material is the same as shown in Figure 5.3 (b).

The simulated and measured results have very similar characteristics from 1 to 9 GHz as shown in Figure 5.13. The simulated S_{11} is mostly under -10 dB from 1.07 to 9 GHz except for the jumps at 4.3, 7 and 8.2 GHz. Compared to this, significant improvement in the impedance matching at these three frequencies is observed in the measured S_{11}. However, the S_{11} at 1.8 GHz, due to the high ε_r of the PEG solution at low frequencies, reaches -6.5 dB.

The simulated maximum gain and penetration efficiency of the antenna are shown in Figure 5.14. The sector-like slot antenna exhibits a slightly higher maximum gain compared to the double-elliptical slot antenna. From 2.5 to 9 GHz, the antenna has a maximum gain almost above 10 dBi. This is due to the fact that the sector-like slot antenna features a larger size in one dimension and thus its directivity increases slightly.

Moreover, the penetration efficiency of the sector-like slot antenna is almost larger than 0.9 (front-to-back ratio of 9.5 dBi). Therefore, the sector-like slot antenna has a slightly better performance in terms of the maximum gain and penetration efficiency.

The simulated and measured near-field patterns (R_{ff}=81.7 mm at 1 GHz, r= 40 mm) of the antenna are shown in Figure 5.15 and 5.16 respectively in the

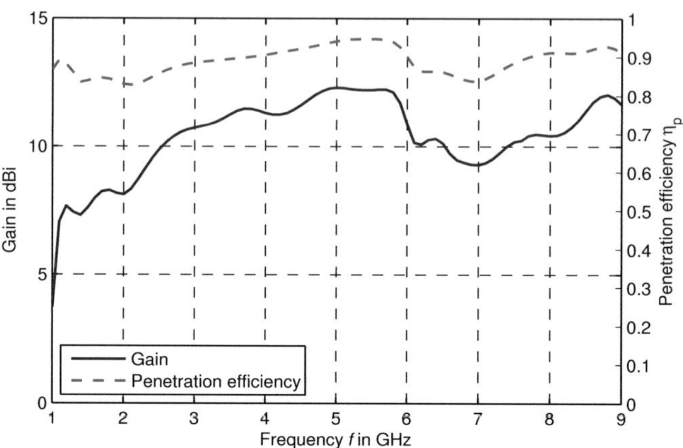

Figure 5.14.: Simulated maximum gain and penetration efficiency of the sector-like slot antenna with the phantom ($\varepsilon_r = 20$, $\sigma = 0$ S/m).

E-plane and H-plane. Slightly asymmetrical patterns at different frequencies are observed and it shows that the asymmetrical connection of radiator and feed network (manufacturing inaccuracy) strongly affect the near-field pattern compared to the double elliptical slot antenna.

The radiation patterns are more directive than those of the double elliptical slot antenna both in the E-plane and H-plane, which is consistent with the simulated maximum gain. The main beam direction in the H-plane is quite constant in the whole frequency band. In the E-plane, the maximum of the pattern at high frequencies is skewed. Significant sidelobes are observed at 4 GHz [Yan11].

Compared to the double-elliptical slot antenna, the lowest operational frequency of the sector-like slot antenna was decreased at the expense of a slightly larger slot size based on the simulated results. However, the measured results exhibited only a slight improvement of the lowest operational frequency, which is strongly affected by the dielectric properties of the tissue-simulating liquid. The final design of the antenna has a size of $35 \times 35 \times 52$ mm^3.

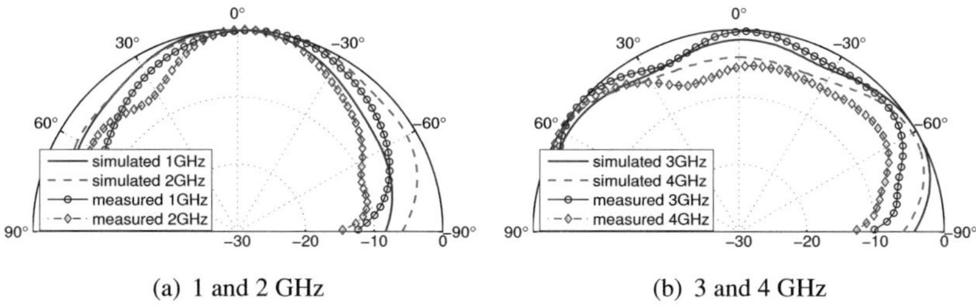

(a) 1 and 2 GHz

(b) 3 and 4 GHz

Figure 5.15.: Simulated and measured near-field pattern of the sector-like slot antenna ($r = 40$ mm), E-plane (yz-plane) for co-polarization (normalized in dB).

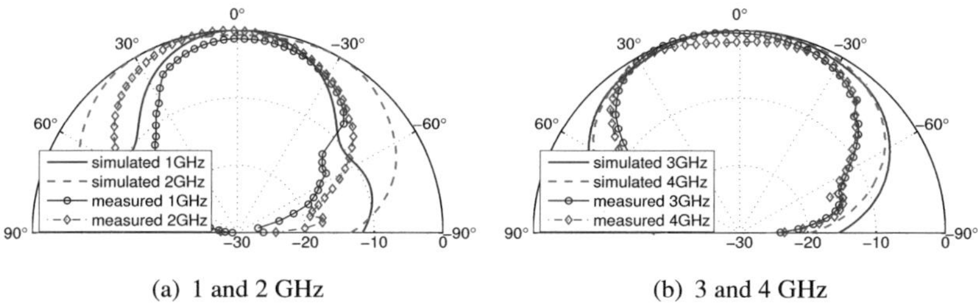

(a) 1 and 2 GHz

(b) 3 and 4 GHz

Figure 5.16.: Simulated and measured near-field pattern of the sector-like slot antenna ($r = 40$ mm), H-plane (xz-plane) for co-polarization (normalized in dB).

5.3.3. Stepped-slot antenna

In order to further lower the lowest operational frequency f_L (by increasing the circumference yet reducing the overall size of the antenna), a stepped-slot design concept is proposed as shown in Figure 5.17. The steps along the whole slot increase the electrical length of the slot. The two steps near the two monopoles allow a good electrical connection between the slot antenna and the feed network. The angles and distances (to the center point of the antenna structure) of the steps are optimized with respect to S_{11} and the radiation pattern [3] [Yan11].

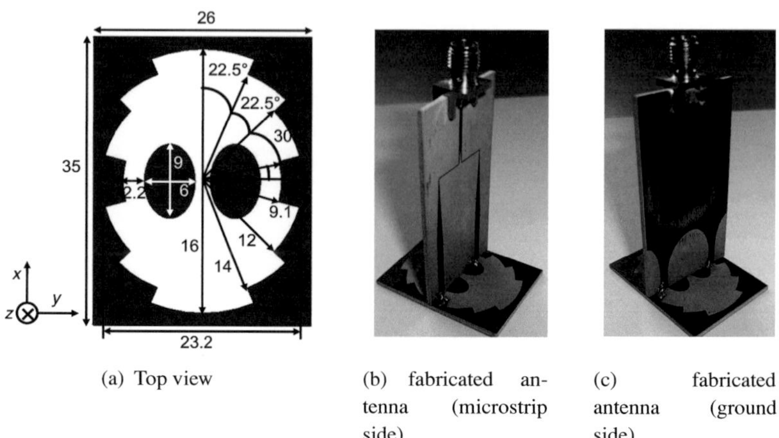

(a) Top view   (b) fabricated antenna (microstrip side)   (c) fabricated antenna (ground side)

Figure 5.17.: Layout and photos of the stepped-slot antenna (conductors are grey, unit: mm).

The sidelobes and grating lobes at high frequencies (especially in the yz-plane) can be minimized by reducing the size of the slot and the distance of the two elliptically shaped monopoles in the y-direction. Furthermore, due to the structure of the stepped-slot, the surface current is concentrated at the edges of the steps (see in Figure 5.18 at different frequencies). Hence the size of the ground area can be significantly reduced (reducing the distance between the slot and the edge of the ground) without influencing the impedance matching of the antenna input port, since the current distribution on the ground at different frequencies is not significantly changed. The final size of the antenna is optimized to be $26{\times}35{\times}52\,\text{mm}^3$.

The S_{11} in Figure 5.19 shows that the simulated antenna is matched to the phantom of the human body from 1 to 9 GHz. The measured result in PEG-water solution shows the S_{11} is under -10 dB in the frequency range from 1.07 to 9 GHz. At high frequencies, a lower S_{11} is observed in the measurement.

The simulated maximal gain of the antenna in contact with the phantom is shown in Figure 5.20. The results show that the antenna has a relatively high and constant gain (> 10 dBi) from 3 to 9 GHz. A small gain is observed at

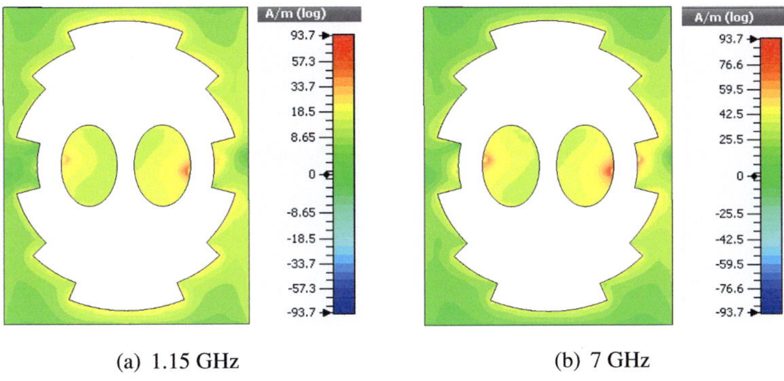

(a) 1.15 GHz   (b) 7 GHz

Figure 5.18.: Surface current distribution of the stepped-slot antenna.

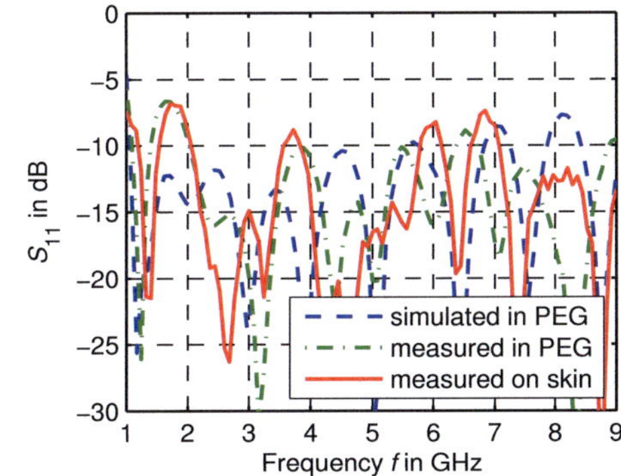

Figure 5.19.: Simulated and measured S_{11} of the stepped-slot antenna over frequency.

the lower frequencies due to the antenna being electrically small in terms of wavelength at the lower frequencies. Moreover, the simulated penetration efficiency confirms that more than 80% of the radiated energy can penetrate into the phantom (human body).

The simulated and measured near-field patterns at a distance of 40 mm from the antenna at different frequencies are shown in Figure 5.21 and 5.22. Symmetrical patterns both in the E-plane and H-plane are observed with a stable

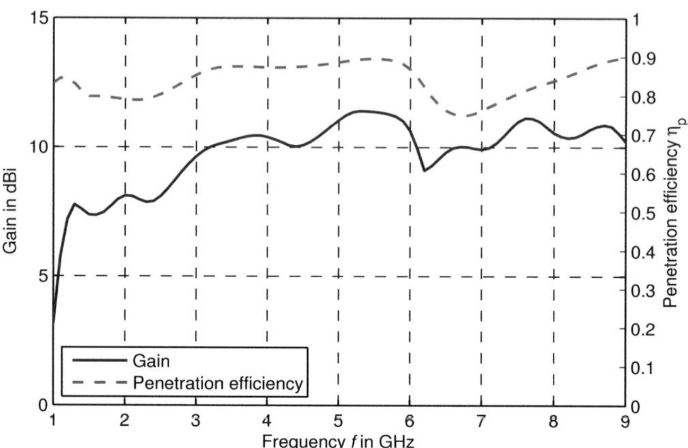

Figure 5.20.: Simulated maximum gain and penetration efficiency of the stepped-slot antenna with the phantom ($\varepsilon_r = 20$, $\sigma = 0$ S/m).

main beam direction due to the phase center being constant over the whole frequency range. It can be seen that the pattern in the E-plane at 3 and 4 GHz features lower sidelobes compared to that of the sector-like slot antenna in Figure 5.15. The reason is that the distance of the two steps (y-direction) near the two monopoles is reduced but the lower frequency is maintained from the miniaturization technique used in this design.

The simulated and experimental results have shown that the stepped-slot antenna is able to radiate in the frequency range from 1 GHz to at least 7 GHz when placed on the human body. The lowest operational frequency of 1.07 GHz is achieved while the antenna size of $26\times35\times52\,\text{mm}^3$ maintains compared to the double-elliptical slot antenna.

5.3.4. Stepped-slot antenna with slotline feed network

After the optimization of the ground of the radiator (the stepped slot), the size of the radiator of $26\times35\,\text{mm}^2$ is obtained. To achieve an even more compact antenna together with a feed network, the feed network must also be miniaturized.

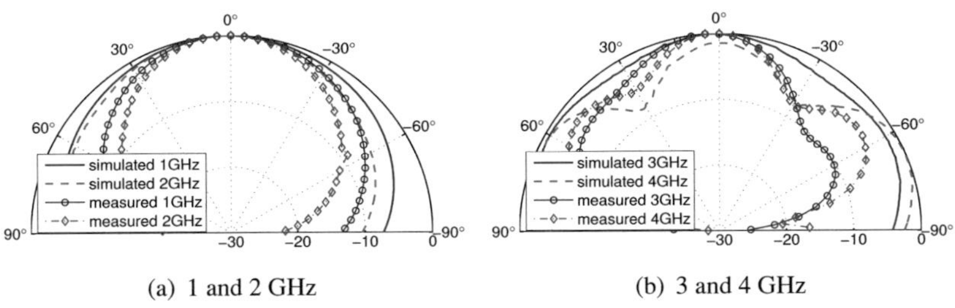

(a) 1 and 2 GHz

(b) 3 and 4 GHz

Figure 5.21.: Simulated and measured near-field pattern of the stepped-slot antenna ($r=$ 40 mm), E-plane (yz-plane) for co-polarization (normalized in dB).

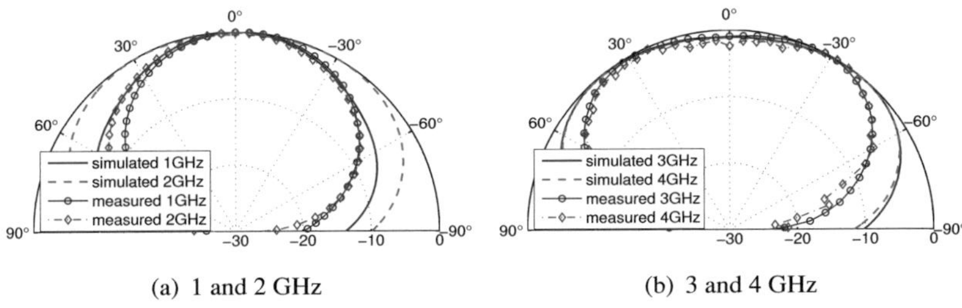

(a) 1 and 2 GHz

(b) 3 and 4 GHz

Figure 5.22.: Simulated and measured near-field pattern of the stepped-slot antenna ($r=$ 40 mm), H-plane (xz-plane) for co-polarization (normalized in dB).

A further size reduction of the feed network using microstrip lines (see in Figure 5.4) is limited by the $\lambda/4$ impedance transformer and tapered ground. Moreover, the connection between the feed network and the radiator introduces further impedance mismatch and loss. Therefore, a new concept of using aperture coupling and a slotline is developed as shown in Figure 5.23. The signal is fed to the microstrip line and transmitted to the slotline through an aperture coupling. The orientation of the E-field along the slotline illustrated in Figure 5.23 (a) causes a differential feed to the monopoles of the radiator. The antenna using this concept is shown in Figure 5.23 (b) and (c).

The Koch-shape (fractal structure) [KGA$^+$09] on the ground plane of the feed network is applied to prevent the radiation of the feed network at the lower frequencies. Since the feed network is connected to the stepped slot radiator, the Koch-shape between the slotlines and monopoles become a loop, which excites unwanted radiation. The direction of this unwanted radiation is normal to the surface of the feed network and the excited frequency is dependent on the circumference of the slot edge. The Koch-shape enables the increase of the circumference within a small area of the ground and hence decrease its resonance frequency down to 1 GHz. A small l_2 and hence small-sized feed network can be achieved.

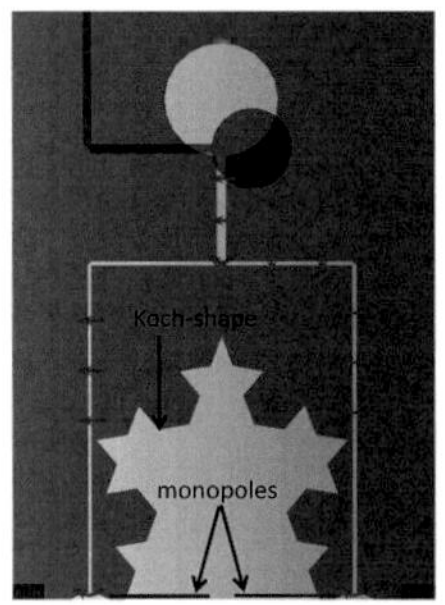

(a) E-field   distribution along the slotline

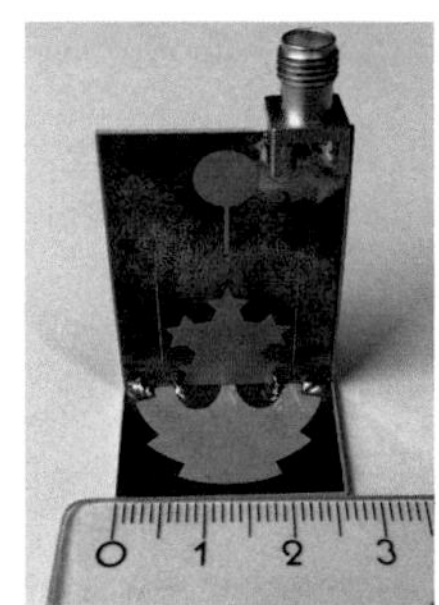

(b) Photo of the antenna (left side)

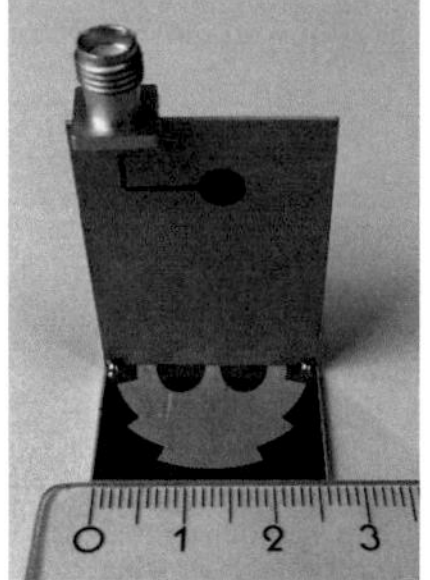

(c) Photo of the antenna (right side)

Figure 5.23.: Design of the stepped slot antenna with the slotline feed network ((a): top and bottom sides superimposed).

The layout of the slotline feed network is shown in Figure 5.24. The rectangular shapes (with dimensions of w_3 and l_3) at the right upper and lower corner on the top side must be soldered together with the slotted ground of the antenna. In this way, the feed network can be fixed stably together with the stepped slot antenna. The width of the slotline on the boundary of the feed network is exactly the same as the distance between monopoles and the slotted ground in the middle of the radiator structure. Therefore, this concept allows for a stable connection between the feed network (slotline) and radiator. The important design parameters are given in Table 5.2.

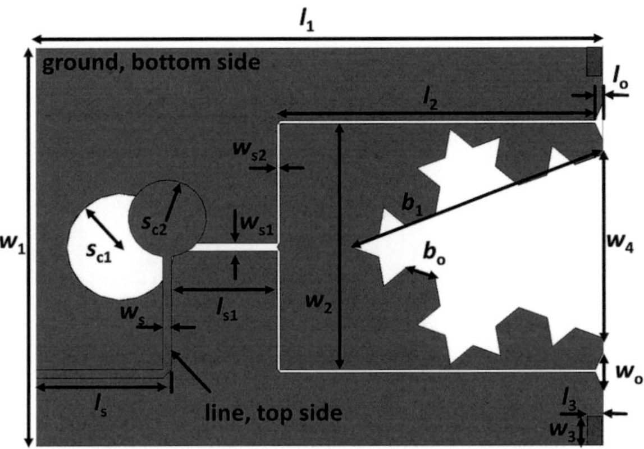

Figure 5.24.: Layout of the slotline feed network (top and bottom sides super-imposed, conductor is grey).

Table 5.2.: Parameters of the slotline feed network.

Parameters	w_1	l_1	w_s	l_s	w_2	l_2	w_3	l_3
Values in mm	26	36.5	0.57	8.79	16.5	20.5	2	1

w_4	w_o	l_o	w_{s1}	w_{s2}	s_{c1}	s_{c2}	b_1	b_o
12	2.5	0.5	0.55	0.2	3.5	2.5	17.35	1.93

From the simulated and measured S_{11} as shown in Figure 5.25, it can be observed that a good impedance matching is achieved from 1 to 7 GHz. The measured result in PEG-water solution shows that the lowest operational frequency is 1.25 GHz, while that of the measurement on the skin is 1.1 GHz. The impedance matching around 7 GHz is about -7.8 dB (measured in PEG-water solution), affected by the impedance matching of the slotline feed network. This is because the slotline feed network exhibits a relatively smaller bandwidth compared with the microstrip feed network (matched from 1 to 10 GHz) [Shu88]. However, the impedance matching of this antenna up to 7 GHz has fulfilled the requirement for microwave medical diagnosis based on the analysis mentioned in chapter 2.

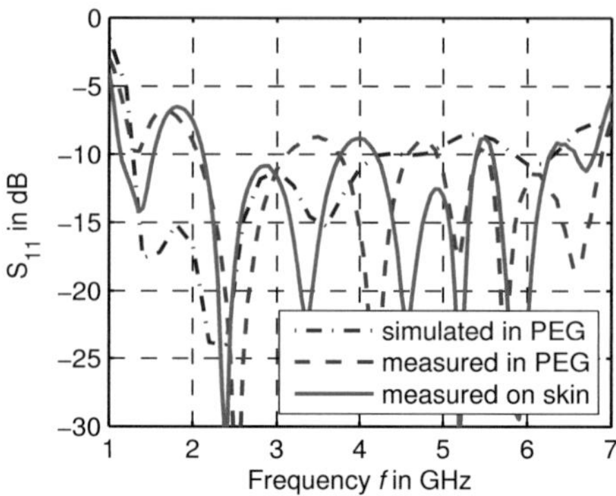

Figure 5.25.: Simulated and measured S_{11} of the stepped slot antenna with slotline feed network over frequency.

Regarding the simulated maximum gain and penetration efficiency shown in Figure 5.26, the antenna features very high gain at the higher frequencies and this drops down significantly at the lower frequencies (about 0 dBi at 1 GHz due to the impedance mismatch). However, the maximum gain at 1.07 GHz is still 2.8 dBi. Similar behavior can be observed with respect to the penetration efficiency. A high front-to-back ratio can be achieved from 3 to 6 GHz, since the penetration depth is larger than 0.9. A minimum of the penetration efficiency (0.65) can be seen at 1.6 GHz. The reason is that the slotline feed network contributes to the radiation into the free space region in this frequency range (from 1.2 to 2.3 GHz). It can be concluded that this antenna has a very high radiation performance in the frequency range from 3 to 7 GHz. The radiation gain and penetration efficiency from 1 to 2 GHz decreased slightly compared to the differentially-fed slot antenna with microstrip feed network. Furthermore, the radiated near-field pattern is verified by comparing the simulated and measured pattern both in the E-plane and H-plane as shown in Figure 5.27 and 5.28, respectively. Compared to the radiation pattern of the stepped-slot antenna with microstrip feed network, the patterns exhibit slightly narrower beamwidth in the E-plane and H-plane.

118

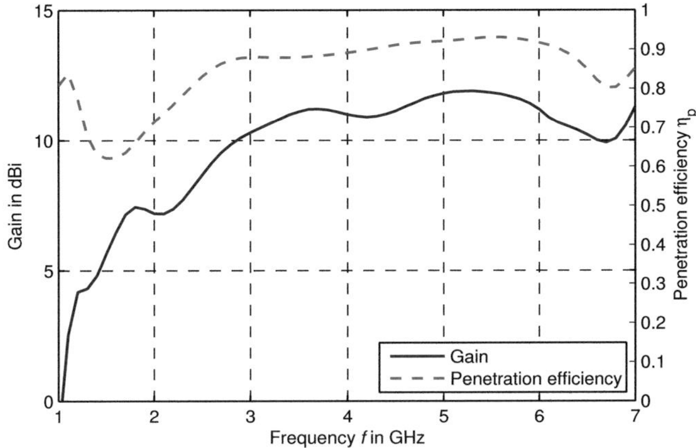

Figure 5.26.: Simulated maximum gain and penetration efficiency of the stepped slot antenna with slotline feed network (phantom: $\varepsilon_r = 20$, $\sigma = 0$ S/m).

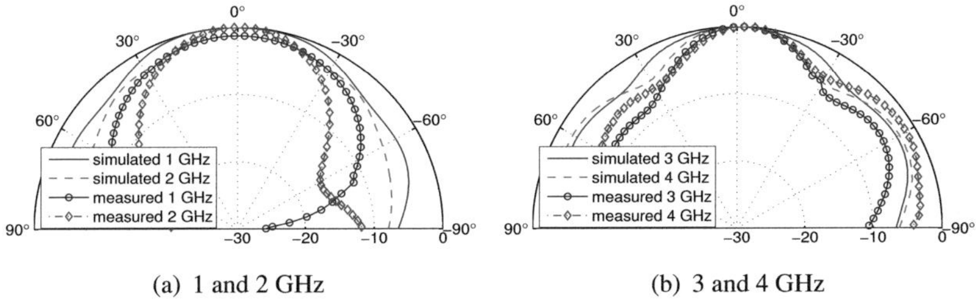

(a) 1 and 2 GHz   (b) 3 and 4 GHz

Figure 5.27.: Simulated and measured near-field pattern of the stepped slot antenna with slotline feed network (r= 40 mm), E-plane (yz-plane) for co-polarization (normalized in dB).

In conclusion, by introducing the new slotline feed network, the antenna size is reduced to $26\times35\times36.5$ mm^3 compared to the antenna with microstrip feed network ($26\times35\times52$ mm^2). The characteristics of the new antenna maintain the desirable operational frequency range from 1 to 7 GHz.

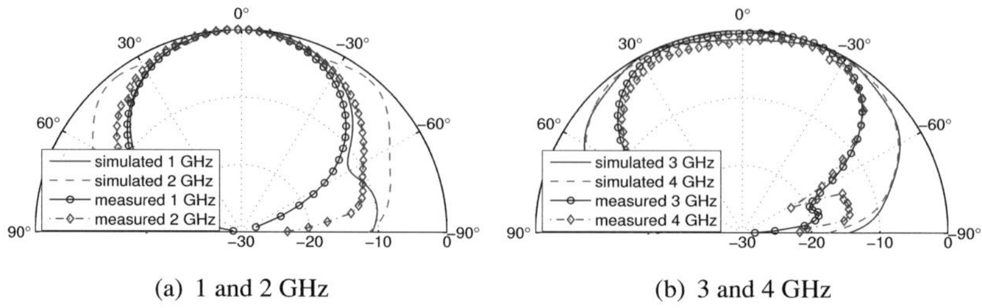

(a) 1 and 2 GHz   (b) 3 and 4 GHz

Figure 5.28.: Simulated and measured near-field pattern of the stepped slot antenna with slotline feed network ($r = 40\,\text{mm}$), H-plane (xz-plane) for co-polarization (normalized in dB).

5.3.5. Summary of the differentially-fed slot antennas

Table 5.3 provides a comparison of the four differentially-fed slot antennas with respect to the size of the antenna together with the feed network, the lowest (f_L) and highest (f_H) operational frequency and the relative bandwidth. Since the impedance matching at the higher frequencies can easily be achieved (even higher than 9 GHz), a stable pattern with low sidelobes is set to be the criterion to determine the highest operational frequency. The upper frequency is based on the simulation results, since the measured pattern is limited up to 4 GHz due to high signal attenuation in tissue-simulating liquid. The lowest operational frequency is determined based on measured S_{11}.

The common ground of the four antennas is that they all have a very stable phase center and a constant main beam direction over the whole operation frequency due to the symmetrical antenna structure. This feature leads to a high applicability of the antenna for pulse-based wideband systems for medical diagnosis. Second, a very high penetration efficiency and front-to-back ratio can be achieved by directly placing the antenna between air and human tissues. This results in a high efficiency of the radiation into the human body and also minimizes the coupling to the environment.

Regarding the size of the radiator, a significant size reduction (26% in one dimension) was successfully achieved by using a stepped slot compared to the sector-like slot. However, increasing the circumference of the slot cannot infinitely decrease the lowest operational frequency. Enlarging the size of the slot can lower the f_L very effectively, but introduces strong sidelobes and grating lobes at high frequencies due to the large size of the slot compared to the wavelength.

The slotline feed network contributed significantly to the size reduction of the overall antenna with feed network. This shows the applicability of the antenna for the construction of antenna arrays within a limited space for medical applications.

The f_L and the operational frequency band of the four antennas show only slight differences. however, the stepped-slot antenna with slotline feed network exhibits the best performance with regard to the impedance matching, the radiation pattern, the size and the robustness.

Table 5.3.: Comparison of the developed differentially-fed slot antennas.

Slot antenna model	Size (mm^3)	f_L (GHz)	f_H (GHz)	Rel. BW
Double-elliptical	26×35×52	1.31	7	137%
Sector-like	35×35×52	1.07	7	147%
Stepped-slot	26×35×52	1.07	7	147%
Stepped-slot with slotline feed network	26×35×36.5	1.1	7	145%

5.4. On-body matched antennas with a lowest operational frequency of 0.5 GHz

In the previous section, different wideband antennas characterized from 1 to 7 GHz were developed, which can be used in radar imaging for medical diagnosis due to the large bandwidth and very low operational frequency. Moreover, the antennas exhibit a robust near-field performance in tissue-simulating liquid. However, to guarantee the deep penetration of the signal inside the head tissues, even lower frequencies ($<$ 1 GHz) are desirable for medical diagnosis (e.g. brain imaging) [17].

In the literature, there are only a few contributions about antennas with very low operational frequency ($< 1\,$GHz) for medical diagnosis. In [TP08], a triangular microstrip antenna with a resonance frequency at $0.7\,$GHz was proposed for stroke detection using an electromagnetic time-domain inversion algorithm. However, the antenna has a large size of $40{\times}46\,$mm^2. A small-sized antenna is regarded as a major challenge for very low operational frequency, since a large number of elements in an array for improving the imaging result are required.

Therefore, the goal of the further antenna development is to design antennas having the lowest operational frequency of $0.5\,$GHz for a deep penetration into human tissues (e.g. brain or heart) and with an antenna size of not larger than $35{\times}35\,$mm^2 (the largest dimensions of the differentially-fed slot antennas). For that reason, two antenna concepts are introduced in the following sections. First, a dual-band slotted Bowtie antenna with microstrip feed and aperture-coupling is described. It is followed by a Bowtie antenna using folded structures with meandered lines and a coaxial-feed. Both of these two antennas provide a lowest operational frequency of about $0.5\,$GHz.

5.4.1. Dual-band aperture-coupled Bowtie antenna

The dual-band aperture-coupled Bowtie antenna has two operational frequency bands, with the first operational band from 0.5 to $0.7\,$GHz (lower frequencies) and the second from 1.3 up to $4\,$GHz (higher frequencies). This antenna is especially suitable for microwave tomography using mono-frequency operation, since the operational frequency can be chosen in different bands.

As shown in Figure 5.29, the dual-band Bowtie antenna consists of a microstrip line as feed on the top side of the substrate and a slotted Bowtie ground plane on the bottom side. The signal is fed by the microstrip line with a characteristic impedance of $50\,\Omega$. The signal is then coupled to the slotline on the bottom side using an aperture-coupled transition. To achieve a broadband transition from microstrip to slotline, the microstrip on the top side is connected to a virtual shorted circular stub [Shu88]. The bandwidth of this transition is determined by the diameter of the circular stub d_{st}, the width of the slot d_{s} and the relative position to the slotline l_{st}. In addition, the photos of the fabricated antenna are shown in Figure 5.30.

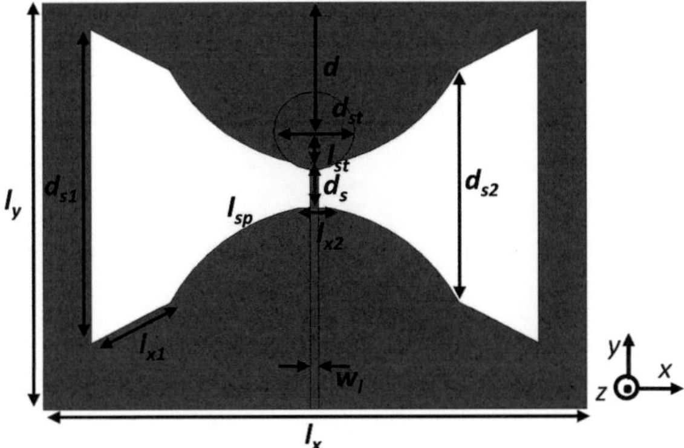

Figure 5.29.: Layout of the dual-band aperture-coupled Bowtie antenna (microstrip line on the top side and slotted Bowtie structure on the bottom side).

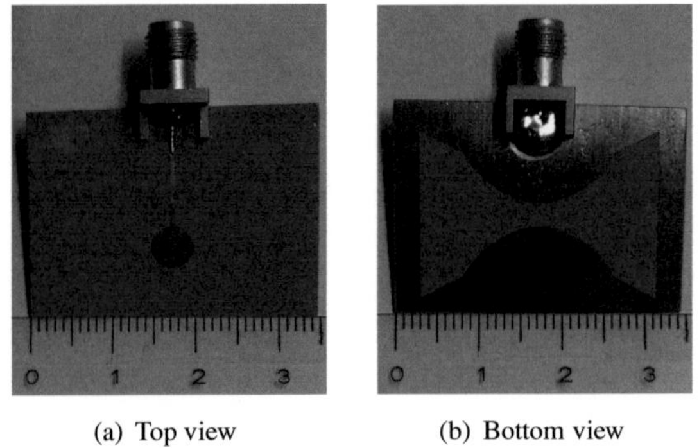

(a) Top view (b) Bottom view

Figure 5.30.: Photos of the fabricated dual-band aperture-coupled Bowtie antenna.

Considering the radiation mechanisms, the EM waves are coupled from the microstrip line to the slotted Bowtie and are radiated. To achieve a broadband impedance matching, the spline curve and the tapered section of the slotted Bowtie are used in addition. Moreover, in Figure 5.31, the E-field distribution between the slotted Bowtie is illustrated, which also indicates the polarization of the radiated waves.

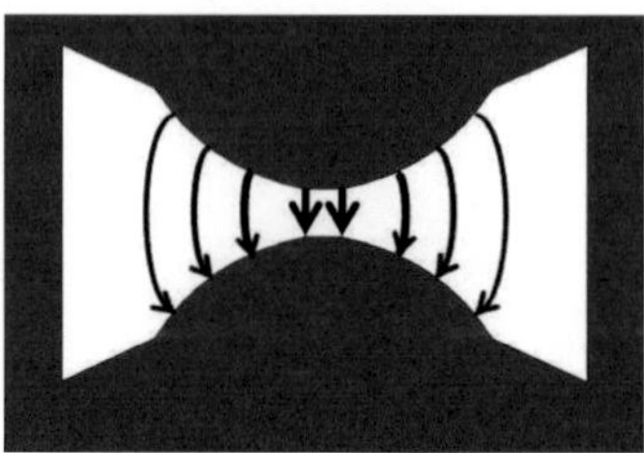

Figure 5.31.: Schematic representation of the E-field distribution between slotted Bowtie of dual-band aperture-coupled Bowtie antenna (dark color denotes the ground of the slot).

Regarding the first operational band, a resonance of the surface current along the slotted Bowtie is excited, which enables the radiation of the E-fields. The central frequency of this band is determined by the circumference of the slot:

$$f_{\mathrm{L}} = \frac{c_0}{C_{\mathrm{s}} \cdot \sqrt{\varepsilon_{\mathrm{r,eff}}}}, \tag{5.4}$$

where C_{s} is the circumference of the slot and is determined as:

$$C_{\mathrm{s}} = 2 \times \left(d_{\mathrm{s1}} + 2l_{\mathrm{x1}} + 2l_{\mathrm{sp}} \right). \tag{5.5}$$

At the second band (high frequencies), the radiation of the traveling waves along the slotted Bowtie occurs. The EM waves propagate from the center point of the slotted Bowtie to the left and right side, respectively. Therefore, the radiations along the slot at the both sides have to be taken into account. With a large aperture of the slot in the x direction, grating lobes at the higher frequencies can be observed. The main pattern in the xz-plane is split into different maximums. This can be minimized by reducing the size of the slot in x-direction. In the optimization procedure, the slot widths (d_{s1} and d_{s2}) are increased in y-direction so that the same circumference for the first band is maintained. In this way, the grating lobes are suppressed at the higher frequencies. The substrate Rogers RT 6010 and thickness of 0.635 mm is chosen for the antenna design and fabrication.

The antenna element is in contact with a phantom material ($\varepsilon_r = 20$ (due to the highest operational frequency up to $4\,\text{GHz}$), $\sigma = 0$ S/m) similar to the different-fed slot antennas in the previous sections. With this configuration, the signals are radiated perpendicularly ($+z$ direction) to the surface of the bottom side of the antenna into the human body. The top side of the antenna is isolated by using an absorber material.

In the parameter optimization, it can be noted that the aperture-coupled transition strongly influences the impedance matching at the two bands, which can be seen in the measured results with varied d_{st} (see Figure 5.32). By tuning d_{st}, an optimal impedance matching can be achieved. The final design parameters of the antenna are given in Table 5.4.

The simulated and measured S_{11} of the slotted Bowtie antenna are shown in Figure 5.33. In the measured S_{11} on skin, the two radiation bands as discussed before can be clearly seen. The measured S_{11} on skin and in PEG-water solution show very similar resonance around $0.55\,\text{GHz}$. However, a slight difference on the whole band is observed due to the multilayer model (skin, fat, muscle), which causes multiple reflections in the measurement on skin. The different resonant frequencies of the measured and simulated S_{11} in PEG-water solution are due to different boundary conditions between simulation and measurement.

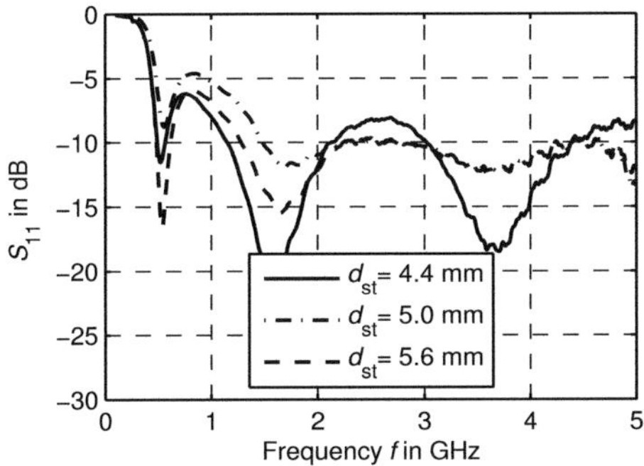

Figure 5.32.: Measured S_{11} of dual-band aperture-coupled Bowtie antenna with different d_{st} on skin.

Table 5.4.: Design parameters of the dual-band aperture-coupled Bowtie antenna.

Parameter	l_x	l_y	d_{s1}	d_{s2}	d_s	l_{x1}
Value (mm)	35	26	20	14.8	2.8	5.6

Parameter	l_{x2}	l_{sp}	w_1	d	d_{st}	l_{st}
Value (mm)	2	11.8	0.52	8.28	5.6	2.1

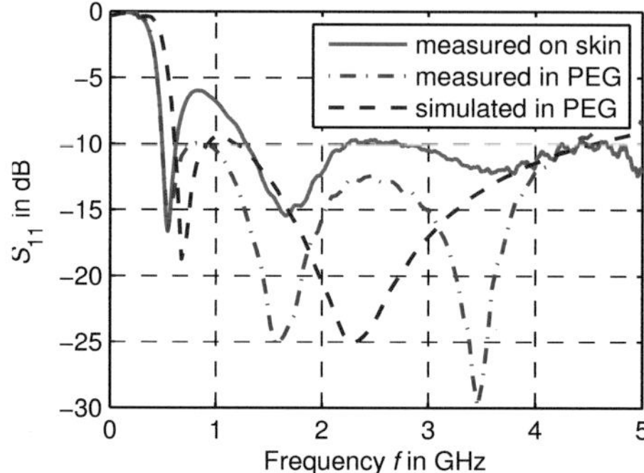

Figure 5.33.: Simulated and measured S_{11} of the dual-band aperture-coupled Bowtie antenna in PEG-water solution and on the skin.

The radiation pattern of the antenna is measured in PEG-water solution at a distance of 5 cm. In the measurement of the radiation pattern, a distance of at least of 5 cm is required to rotate the AUT in the E-plane by 180°, since the feed point of the antenna is at the side of the substrate (refer to Figure 5.30) and hence additional space is needed for the connector. This distance (5 cm) corresponds to the radiating near-field region of the antenna at the second band (1.3 to 4 GHz), but the far-field region at the first band (0.5 to 0.7 GHz). The measured radiation pattern is limited to 2 GHz with a measurement distance of 5 cm to the antenna. As shown in Figure 5.34, the measured pattern in the E-plane is asymmetrical. This is because the current distribution of the slotted Bowtie is asymmetrical due to the feed being on one side of the ground. However, the main beam direction remains normal to the surface of the antenna. In the H-plane, the patterns are very similar at 0.6 GHz, 1 GHz and 2 GHz.

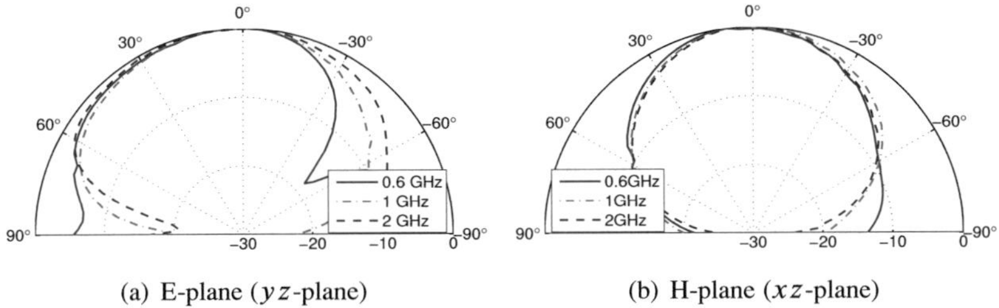

(a) E-plane (yz-plane) (b) H-plane (xz-plane)

Figure 5.34.: Measured radiation pattern of dual-band aperture-coupled Bowtie antenna ($r = 50\,$mm), in co-polarization (normalized in dB).

In conclusion, the dual-band slotted Bowtie antenna features an extremely small size of $34{\times}26\,$mm^2. The antenna can be operated in the frequency range from 0.5 to 0.7 GHz and from 1.3 to 4 GHz.

This antenna is suitable for microwave tomography systems, in which mono-frequency operation at different frequencies are required to be evaluated. Operating from 0.5 to 4 GHz for radar imaging for medical diagnosis, the antenna can introduce additional signal distortion (e.g. signal in the time domain), since the stop band from 0.7 to 1.3 GHz exists. In the next section, an optimized Bowtie antenna characterized from 0.5 GHz to at least 2 GHz is described for the radar imaging for medical diagnosis.

5.4.2. Compact double-layer folded Bowtie antenna

A regular Bowtie antenna is preferred for the design of UWB antennas in free space, since it features wideband impedance matching and low design complexity. Matching the regular Bowtie antenna to the human body with the lowest operational frequency at 0.5 GHz, the Bowtie antenna will have a size of at least $50 \times 50\,$mm^2 using the substrate RT 6010 (thickness of 1.27 mm). Therefore, the miniaturization of the regular Bowtie antenna is the focus of this section.

The miniaturization technique of the regular Bowtie antenna by the optimization of its structure is used. The main idea is to increase the current path along the antenna to fulfill the radiation requirements and maintain the antenna size. Based on this, a compact double-layer folded Bowtie antenna is developed and described in the following paragraphs.

To maintain a realistic scenario, a phantom emulating the human body is placed on the bottom side of the antenna in the simulation as shown in Figure 5.35. The phantom (ε_r=35, σ=0 S/m) has the average relative permittivity of skin and fat at 0.5 GHz [GGC96, GLG96a, GLG96b] and the dispersion of the phantom material is not considered in the primary optimization of the antenna based on the design principle discussed at the beginning of the chapter. At the top side of the antenna, the free space region is maintained. The direction of the radiation is normal to the planar surface of the antenna and goes into the phantom.

To miniaturize the Bowtie antenna, a new concept by the introduction of a double-layer structure and meandered lines is proposed. The antenna consisting of two identical substrates is shown in Figure 5.36. Structure 1 is the Bowtie element on the bottom side of the antenna, which is folded and connected together with two symmetric meandered lines at the top side of the antenna. With this concept, at low frequencies, the antenna acts like a closed loop consisting of the Bowtie and the meandered lines. The electrical length at the lower frequencies is enlarged by the meandered line hence the size of the antenna can be significantly reduced. Looking at a superimposed image of structure 1 and 3, the meandered structure must not overlap the triangles, which make up the Bowtie antenna to ensure that the radiation is normal to the antenna surface. Furthermore, the resonance between the Bowtie structure and the meandered lines can be prevented in this way and wideband operation of the antenna is then guaranteed. At the higher frequencies, the radiation is mainly based on the Bowtie structure. A good impedance matching for a high efficiency of radiation for the whole frequency range is thus required and is done by optimizing the parameters of structure 1 and 3.

A coaxial cable (shown in Figure 5.36 (d)) with an inner diameter of 0.9 mm and an outer diameter of 3.0 mm (characteristic impedance: 50 Ω) is used to connect to the antenna structure normally to the top side of the antenna. A

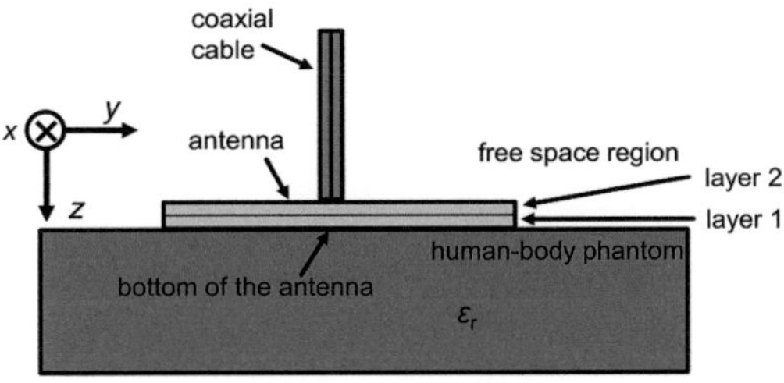

Figure 5.35.: Arrangement of the double-layer folded Bowtie antenna together with the phantom.

balun (on structure 2 and 3) using a microstrip line is used to convert the un-
balanced coaxial feed to symmetrical (balanced) feed for the Bowtie structure.
The inner conductor of the coaxial cable is connected through the microstrip
on structure 2 to the left triangle on structure 1, while the outer conductor of
coaxial cable is connected to the right triangle. Two vias allow the connection
between different structures.

Regarding the current distribution as shown in Figure 5.37, a strong current
exists around the two feed points on the Bowtie structure and flows further
to the two sides. At 0.5 GHz (lower frequency) the current is concentrated
along the meandered line at the top side. A long electrical length at this
frequency can clearly be identified. At the higher frequencies (e.g. 1.5 GHz),
as expected in the analysis, the current flows along the Bowtie structure with
higher intensity and lower current density on the meandered line is observed,
which results in a low influence of the meandered structure with regard to the
impedance matching at high frequencies [Bar12].

Details of the parameter study regarding the impedance matching are described in the following paragraphs. All relevant parameters are shown in
Figure 5.36. Increasing w_1, the impedance matching at high frequencies is
improved and hence the bandwidth of the antenna is increased significantly
(see in Figure 5.38 (a)). However, the S_{11} degrades at the higher frequencies when the value of w_1 becomes too large (e.g. 14.8 mm) due to the bad
impedance matching at the feed points of the Bowtie structure. Furthermore,

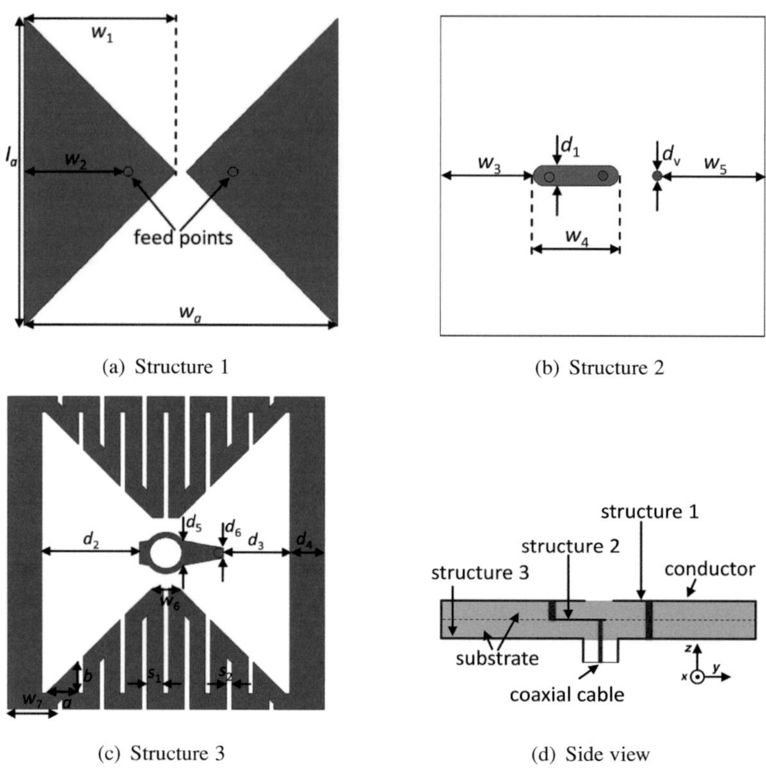

Figure 5.36.: The layout of the doubled-layered Bowtie antenna.

only slight changes of the lowest operational frequency (determined by S_{11} below -10 dB) of the antenna with varied w_1 are observed.

The input impedance of the Bowtie structure is dependent on the position of its feed point (w_2), which allows the impedance matching from the coaxial cable to the Bowtie structure. Figure 5.38 (b) shows the reflection coefficient at the coaxial port of the antenna with different w_2. It must be noted that the impedance matching at the lower frequencies is almost independent of w_2. However, the S_{11} degrades at the higher frequencies with increasing w_2. At w_2=14 mm, a bandwidth of 1 GHz (from 0.45 to 1.45 GHz) is observed. This

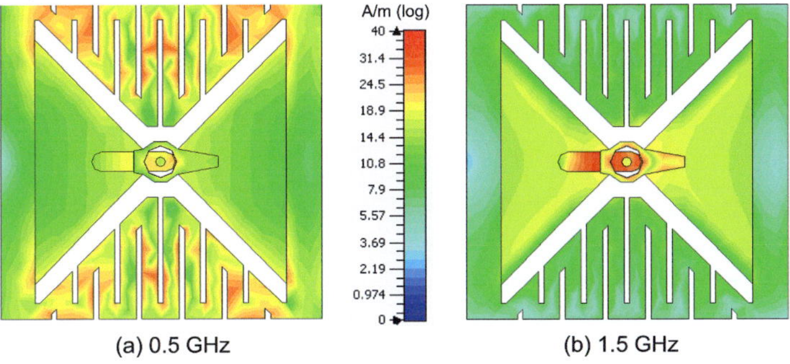

Figure 5.37.: Surface current distribution of the doubled-layered Bowtie antenna at 0.5 GHz and 1.5 GHz(overlapping of three layers).

is because the feed points are too close to the middle of the Bowtie structure resulting in very high input impedance between the two feed points at the higher frequencies. The impedance mismatch is caused by the connection at the higher frequencies from the coaxial cable to the Bowtie structure by vias.

Since the antenna is matched to the human skin and the dielectric property of human skin differ among people, the sensitivity of the antenna to the permittivity of the human skin is investigated. The simulations are performed with 4 different permittivities of the phantom (see Figure 5.35). The simulated S_{11} in Figure 5.39 shows that the curves shift slightly to the low frequency region with higher permittivity of phantom since the wavelength in the phantom with high relative permittivity becomes smaller. The frequency shift at the lowest operating frequency is weaker than that at the highest operating frequency. This is due to the current distribution on the meandered line, which mostly contributes to the radiation at low frequencies, being not strongly affected by the change of the relative permittivity of the phantom. Furthermore, the bandwidth remains almost the same. Therefore, it can be concluded that the impedance matching of the antenna is not degraded strongly, when the dielectric property of human skin changes slightly. Therefore, the antenna shows low sensitivity to the permittivity of human skin and is applicable for diagnostics on different parts of human body or different patients.

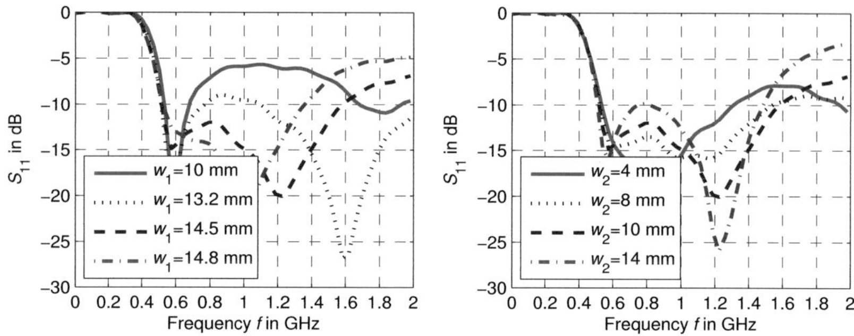

Figure 5.38.: Simulated S_{11} of the double-layer folded Bowtie antenna with different widths w_1 and w_2.

For the purpose of the comparison with regard to the size reduction, the double-layer folded Bowtie antenna and a reference antenna (regular Bowtie antenna) are shown in Figure 5.40. The designs of these antennas having the same operational frequency band (0.5 to 2 GHz in this work) are based on the configuration shown in Figure 5.35.

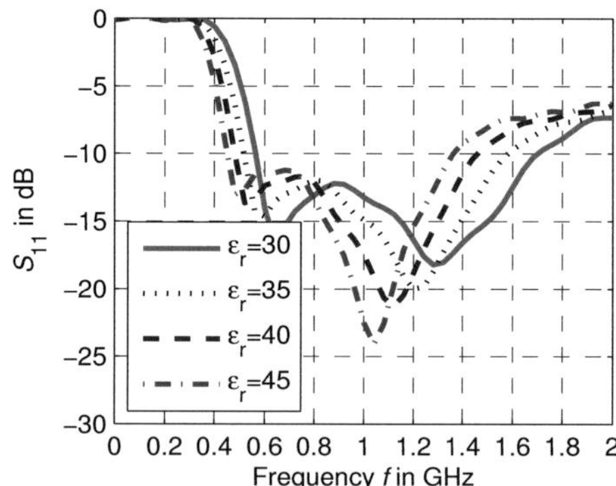

Figure 5.39.: Simulated S_{11} of the proposed antenna with different Permittivities (ϵ_r) of the phantom (σ=0 S/m).

The optimization of the antenna is performed by adjusting all parameters accordingly. Finally, the simulated S_{11} of the proposed antenna and the reference antenna are provided in Figure 5.41. These two antennas indicate similar operational bandwidth, especially at the same lowest operational frequency of 0.5 GHz. However, the size of the proposed antenna ($30 \times 30\,\mathrm{mm}^2$) is reduced by 40 % compared to the reference antenna ($50 \times 50\,\mathrm{mm}^2$).

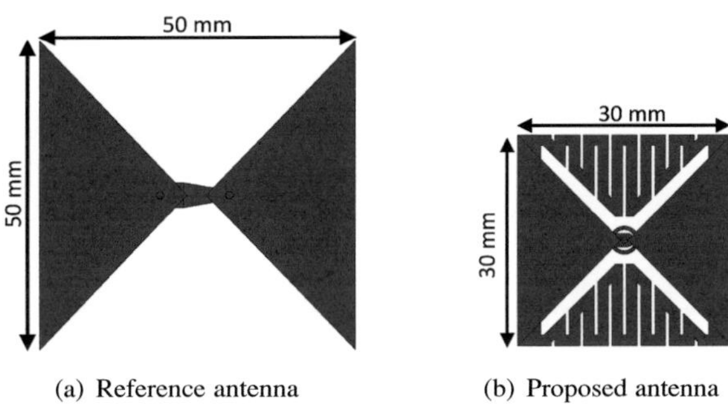

Figure 5.40.: Layout of the reference antenna (regular Bowtie antenna) and the doubled-layer Bowtie antenna.

After the initial optimization of the antenna with the phantom (ε_r=35, σ=0 S/m), a further optimization of the antenna is performed using realistic dielectric properties (PEG-water solution) to include the conductivity and frequency dispersion. The final optimized parameters of the antenna are given in Table 5.5. The size of the optimized antenna ($30 \times 30\,\mathrm{mm}^2$) remains.

The fabricated antenna is shown in Figure 5.42. Figure 5.43 shows the simulated S_{11} in PEG and the measured S_{11} in PEG-water solution and on human skin. The antenna is finally optimized in PEG-water solution with S_{11} below -10 dB from 0.5 to 2 GHz with a relative bandwidth of 120 %.

The simulated and measured results in PEG-water solution have very similar run of the curves. The simulated S_{11} is below -10 dB in the whole frequency range from 0.5 to 2 GHz, while the measured S_{11} indicates a slightly lower operational frequency of 0.45 GHz. The difference at around 1 GHz of S_{11} could be caused by leaking of PEG-water solution into the free space region at the top of the antenna. However, this problem can be avoided in a real

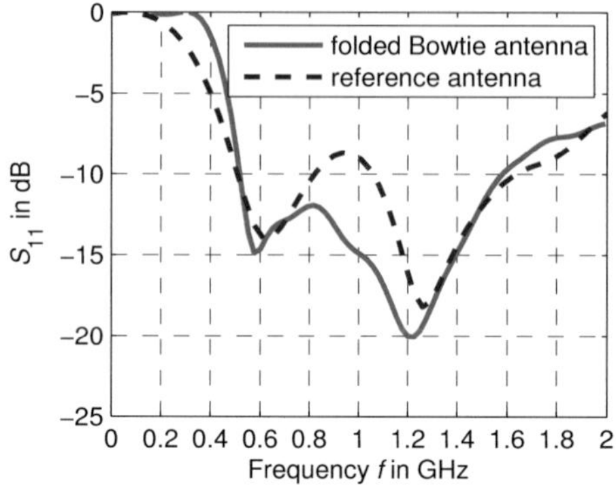

Figure 5.41.: Simulated S_{11} of the proposed antenna and the reference antenna with the phantom (ϵ_r=35, σ=0 S/m).

Table 5.5.: Parameters of the antenna

Parameter	Value (mm)	Parameter	Value (mm)
w_a	30	d_2	9.56
l_a	30	d_3	6.3
w_1	14.5	d_4	3.25
w_2	9.56	d_5	2.4
w_3	8.61	d_6	1
w_4	7.8	w_6	2.52
d_v	0.9	s_1	1.5
d_1	1.9	s_2	0.5
w_5	9.56	a	3.11
d_2	9.3	b	3.11

measurement scenario on the human body, since the antennas are in contact with the human body and tissue-simulating liquid is not required.

The measured S_{11} on the human skin shows a better S_{11} in a realistic scenario. Two very strong resonances can be observed due to the presence of multi-reflections between the multilayer tissues. The S_{11} of -10 dB, ranging from 0.44 GHz to at least 2 GHz, shows a bandwidth of more than 1.5 GHz.

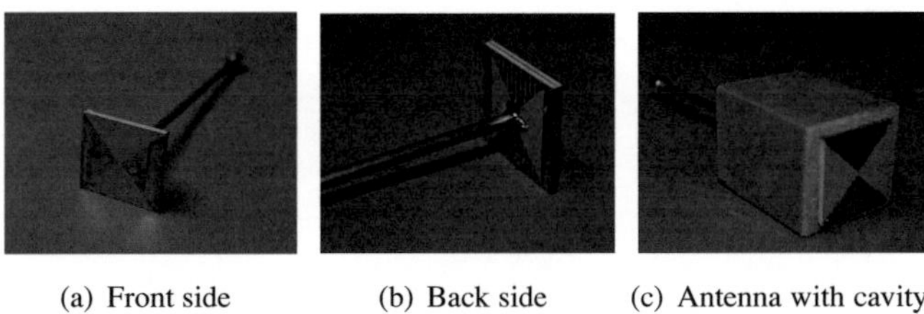

(a) Front side   (b) Back side   (c) Antenna with cavity

Figure 5.42.: Photos of the fabricated antenna with coaxial cable and cavity of Styrofoam.

Considering the different arrangement of the double-layer folded Bowtie antenna (radiator placed between the substrate and the human body) compared to the differentially-fed slot antenna (radiator placed between the substrate and free space region), the penetration efficiency of the double-layer folded Bowtie antenna is investigated. The results in Figure 5.44 show that the penetration efficiency almost remains the same with the increase of the relative permittivity of the phantom (ε_r) at the higher frequencies (from 1.25 to 2 GHz). However, at the lower frequencies, the penetration efficiency is improved with increased ε_r. The reason is that, at the lower frequencies, the current distribution of the whole antenna can be significantly altered due to the presence of the meandered lines (at the top side of the antenna) by the changing contrast of the permittivities between the phantom and air. In the case of lower ε_r (e.g. 20), significant radiation into free space from the meandered lines at the top side of the antenna occurs. With higher ε_r (e.g. 35), more electric fields (more than 75% at 0.5 GHz) are radiated into the phantom because of a longer electrical length of the Bowtie structures at the bottom side of the antenna leading to a larger effective wavelength. Therefore, the radiation from the Bowtie structures into the phantom increases. In Figure 5.45, it can be seen that a η_p of 0.9 can be achieved in the frequency range from 1 to 2 GHz. This corresponds to a extremely high front-to-back ratio (9.5 dB). The simulated maximal gain of the antenna in the main beam direction with the phantom (ε_r=35, σ=0 S/m) is shown in Figure 5.45. The results show that the antenna has a relatively high and constant gain ($\geq$ 6 dBi) from 1 to 2 GHz. A small gain is observed at the lower frequencies compared to the gain at the

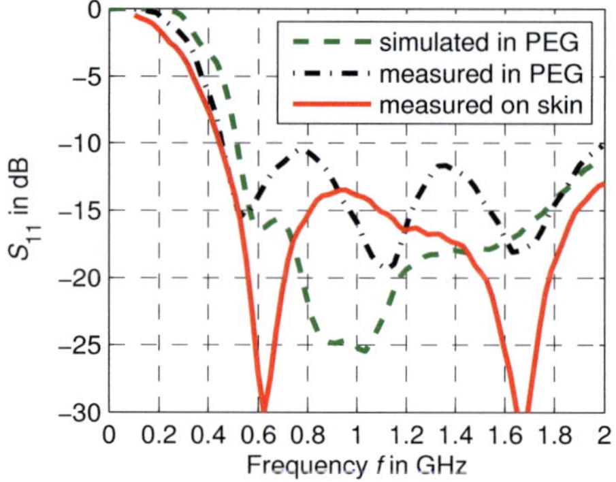

Figure 5.43.: Simulated and measured S_{11} of the double-layer folded Bowtie antenna.

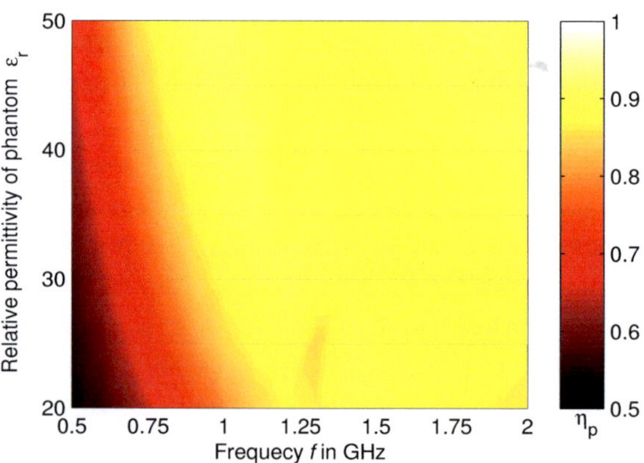

Figure 5.44.: Simulated penetration efficiency η_p (in linear scale) of the double-layer folded Bowtie antenna over frequency with varied relative permittivity ε_r of phantom (σ =0 S/m).

high frequencies. At 2 GHz, a decrease of the gain is observed. It is because that the balun for the connection of the cable and Bowtie structure causes loss at the higher frequencies due to the presence of surface waves and high mode of the propagating waves. It can be still concluded that the antenna features a very high radiation gain and radiation efficiency (better than 91% on the whole operational band neglecting the conductivity of the phantom).

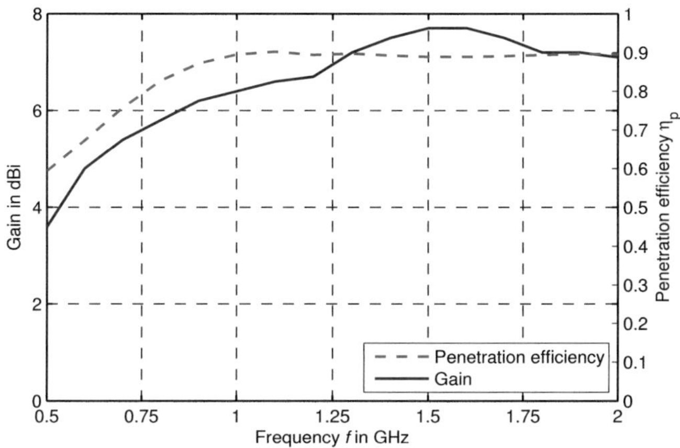

Figure 5.45.: Simulated gain and penetration efficiency of the double-layer folded Bowtie antenna ($\varepsilon_r = 35$, σ =0 S/m).

The simulated and measured radiation pattern at different frequencies (0.5, 1, 1.5 and 2 GHz) are shown in Figure 5.46 and 5.47 in the E-plane and H-plane, respectively. The measurements are performed in the PEG-water solution and the E-fields of the radiation are captured at a distance of 50 mm from the antenna. As discussed in dual-band aperture-coupled Bowtie antenna, it must be emphasized that the near-field region cannot be maintained for the whole frequency range due to the geometric limitation in the measurement (rotation of the AUT required). The measurement distance of 50 mm is far-field region at 0.5 GHz (R_{ff}=71 mm), which the radiating near-field pattern can be measured at this distance at 1 GHz (R_{ff}=35.5 mm). A symmetrical pattern at different frequencies is observed due to the symmetrical antenna

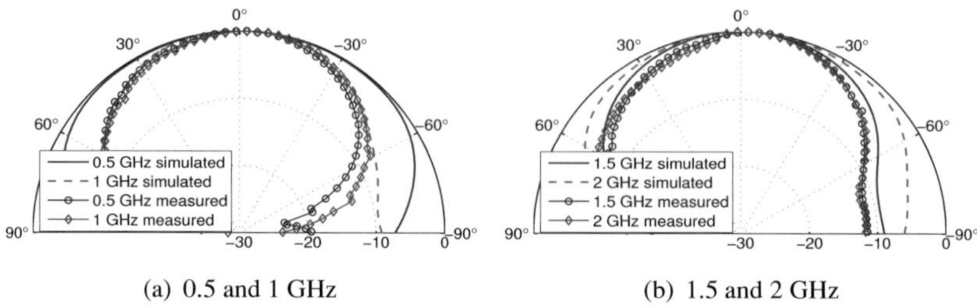

(a) 0.5 and 1 GHz

(b) 1.5 and 2 GHz

Figure 5.46.: Simulated and measured radiation pattern of the double-layer folded Bowtie antenna ($r = 50\,\text{mm}$), E-plane (yz-plane) for co-polarization (normalized in dB).

and feeding structures. In the E-plane, minor sidelobes can be seen. The beamwidth in the H-plane is wider than in the E-plane and the pattern are very similar at different frequencies.

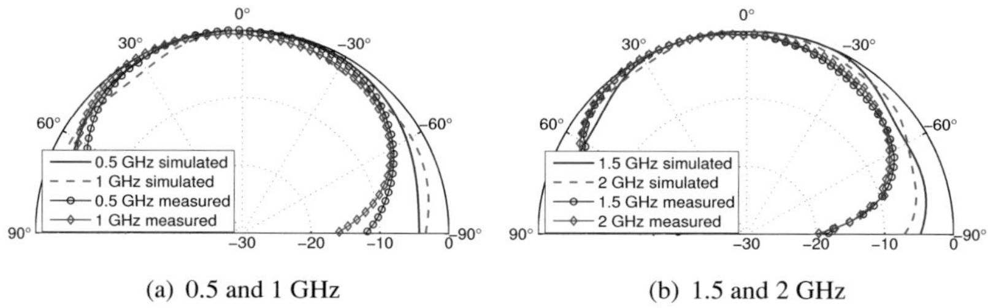

(a) 0.5 and 1 GHz

(b) 1.5 and 2 GHz

Figure 5.47.: Simulated and measured radiation pattern of the double-layer folded Bowtie antenna ($r = 50\,\text{mm}$), H-plane (xz-plane) for co-polarization (normalized in dB).

The SAR value is investigated in simulation of the antenna together with a head model (shown in Figure 5.48). The frequency dependent dielectric properties including conductivity of the tissues are taken into account (according to [GLG96a][GLG96b]). The head model consists of skin, skull, grey matter and white matter with a dimension of $60 \times 60\,\text{mm}^2$ in the cross section (xy-plane).

The radiated E-fields in different tissues in the simulation are recorded and the corresponding SAR values are calculated by (3.11). The density of different tissues according to [BBH70] are used. As results, the 10 g averaged SAR distribution of the cross section in skin and grey matter are depicted in Figure 5.49 and 5.50 at different frequencies, respectively. The input power of 1 mW is used to calculate the SAR.

As can be seen in these results, the distributions at different frequencies are similar but however with different intensity. At the higher frequencies (e.g. 2 GHz), the SAR values are higher than at the lower frequencies. This is due to the higher penetration efficiency and gain at the higher frequencies, which result in stronger E-fields in tissues. Moreover, a large conductivity also contributes to higher SAR values at the higher frequencies. In the grey matter, the SAR values decrease compared to in the skin layer, since the E-fields are attenuated during the propagation from the skin to grey matter. Overall, the maximum value in the model is 0.06 W/kg (10 g tissue), which fulfills the requirements for general public exposure according to [oNiRPI98, Com01, CLC95].

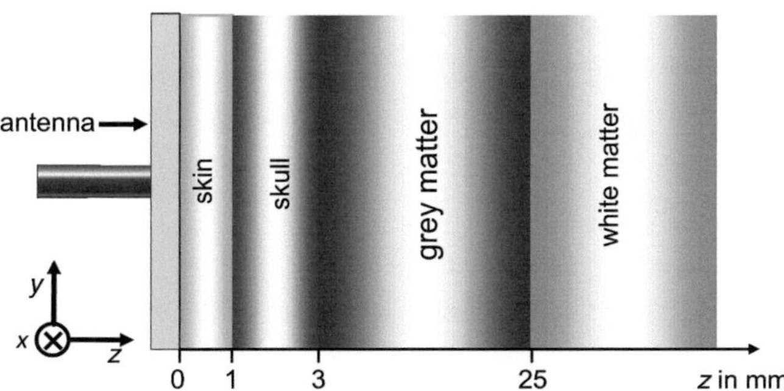

Figure 5.48.: Simulation model of the human head with the double-layer folded Bowtie antenna for evaluation of the SAR.

It can be concluded that the design of the double-layer on-body matched antenna using the folded-Bowtie and meandered lines allows a significant miniaturization of the antenna size. The radiation mechanism is validated

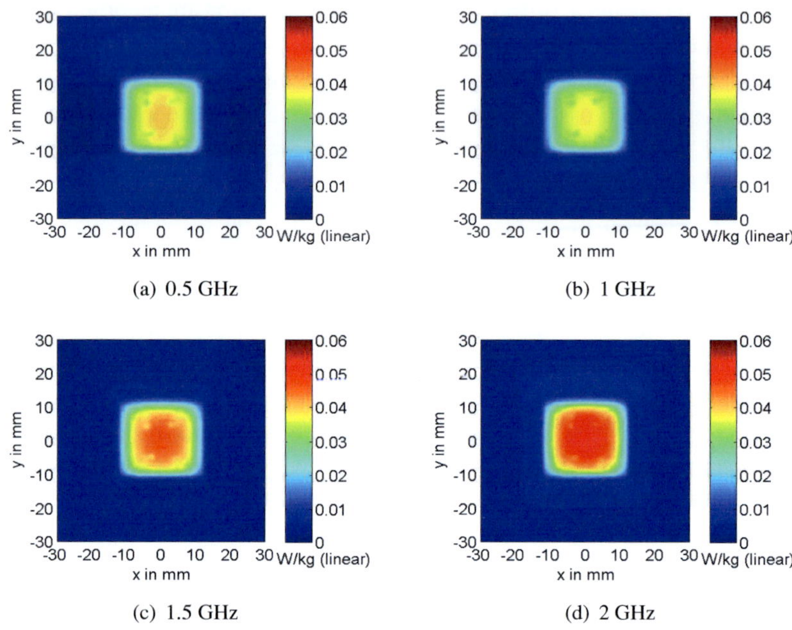

Figure 5.49.: Simulated SAR distributions in the human head for an input power of 1 mW: slices of SAR at $z = 0.5\,\mathrm{mm}$ in the skin layer.

by observing the current distribution at different frequencies. The parameter study showed that the impedance matching at the lower frequencies is strongly dependent on the meandered structure at the top side, while the size of the Bowtie structure and the feeding position affect the performance at the higher frequencies. The final design after parameter optimization is characterized from 0.5 to 2 GHz and enables a size reduction of 40% compared to the reference antenna (regular Bowtie antenna). The simulation results are validated with a special measurement system using the tissue-simulating liquid (PEG-water solution). The measured results agree well with the simulation results. Moreover, the investigation of the SAR based on a multilayer model of the human head showed the applicability of the proposed antenna for medical diagnosis (e.g. stroke detection). The antenna characteristics such as

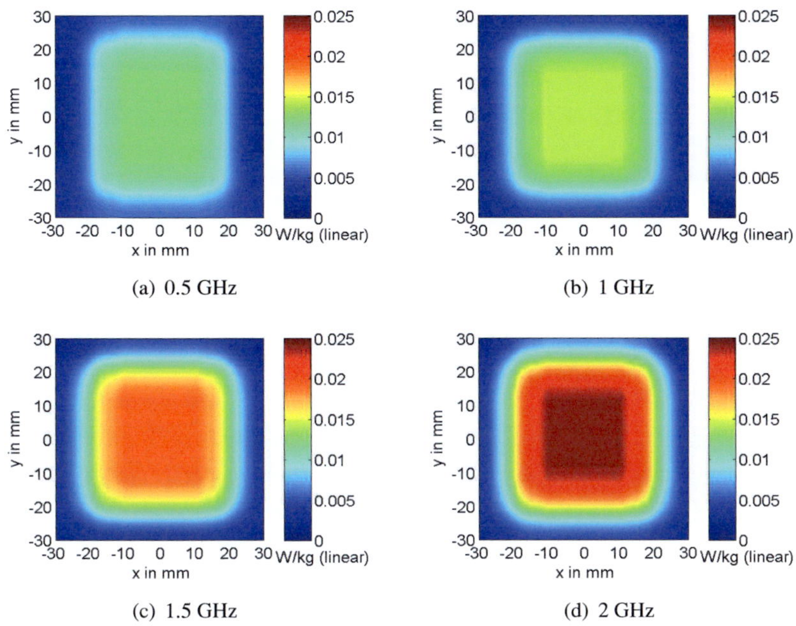

Figure 5.50.: Simulated SAR distributions in the human head for an input power of 1 mW: slices of SAR at $z = 5\,\text{mm}$ in the grey matter layer.

high gain, efficiency and front-to-back ratio will improve the SNR of radar imaging system.

5.5. Summary

In reviewing the design challenges of on-body matched antennas, the general design principles of these antennas were established with the aid of promoting the optimization procedures and guaranteeing the simulation accuracy. The efficiency of the proposed design procedure for on-body matched antenna is reflected significantly in the development of the proposed antennas in this

Table 5.6.: Overview of the developed on-body matched antennas in this chapter (measured results).

Antenna model	Size (mm^2)	Frequency band (GHz)	Rel. BW
Double-elliptical slot	26×35	1.31-7	137%
Sector-like slot	35×35	1.07-7	147%
Stepped-slot	26×35	1.07-7	147%
Stepped-slot with slotline feed network	26×35	1.1-7	145%
Dual-band Bowtie	26×35	0.5-0.7 and 1.3-4	-
Double-layer Bowtie	30×30	0.44 - 2	128%

chapter.

A short overview of the developed on-body matched antennas are given in Table 5.6 with respect to the different characteristics in simulation and measurement. Regarding the operational frequency band, the developed antennas can be divided into two categories. The differentially-fed slot antennas belong to the first category, which exhibits impedance matching in the frequency range from around 1 to 7 GHz. These antennas can be used for microwave medical imaging, where high range resolution and hence a large bandwidth are desirable. The studies of different concepts of slotted ground and feed networks showed that the lowest operational frequency was improved slightly. However, the size reduction of the antenna was of great significance for the overall size and performance of the imaging system based on these antennas.

All of these four slot antennas indicated a stable phase center over the whole operated frequency range and a high front-to-back ratio. Among these, the stepped-slot antenna with slotline feed network features the smallest antenna size ($26×35×36.5\,mm^3$) and lowest operational frequency of 1.1 GHz, which shows a high potential for medical imaging systems (e.g. radar imaging) for the detection of breast cancer, stroke in human brain and other relevant medical diagnosis.

For a deeper penetration of EM waves into human tissues (e.g. brain or heart), two modified Bowtie antennas with a lowest operational frequency of 0.5 GHz were designed. The dual-band aperture coupled Bowtie antenna allows to perform microwave imaging diagnosis in different frequency bands using microwave tomography. For the usage of the whole frequency band from 0.5 GHz to at least 2 GHz, a double-layer folded Bowtie antenna can be used.

All of the antennas proposed in this chapter were significantly miniaturized based on different techniques. In this way, more antenna elements can be implemented in an array within a limited area/space for medical diagnosis and therefore, more data can be gathered from medical scenarios. This small-sized antenna, will contribute positively to the improvement of the resolution and signal-to-clutter ratio (SCR) of microwave imaging systems for medical diagnosis such as stroke and breast cancer detection.

To demonstrate the applicability of the proposed antennas, an antenna array with the stepped-slot antenna with slotline feed network is constructed and a microwave imaging system together with a brain phantom will be discussed in the following chapter.

6. Body-matched antennas based microwave medical imaging

In the previous chapters, various designs of body-matched antennas were developed for different operational frequency bands and radiation properties. To demonstrate the performance enhancement of microwave medical systems utilizing the designed body-matched antennas, this chapter provides a feasibility study of the microwave medical diagnosis for stroke detection by using a realistic measurement setup.

The measurement setup using the on-body matched antennas is demonstrated for a comparison with the system using the off-body antennas. Investigations by the author in [20] [Riv11] showed that the detection of water accumulation in an oil-phantom with Vivaldi-antennas (matched in free space) was not successful. The reason is that there is a strong reflection from the air-phantom interface and strong antenna coupling, which cannot be strictly calibrated from the received signals. Thus, the detection capability and imaging results of the microwave medical imaging system is significantly degraded. Therefore, the goal of this chapter is to show the impact of the developed on-body matched antennas on the system performance. These antennas feature a very low operational frequency (about 1 GHz), stable radiation pattern and compact size of a single antenna, which improves the penetration capability and image quality (contrast, resolution and signal-to-clutter ratio (SCR)) of the microwave medical imaging system.

In the first section, the measurement setup together with a brain phantom for the hemorrhagic stroke detection is introduced. Next, the calibration methods for removing the background reflection and antenna coupling as well as the applied imaging algorithm (wideband beamforming algorithm based on time-domain signals) are presented. The received signals are then analyzed and the results of the two-dimensional (2D) microwave imaging are provided.

Finally, the improvements of the on-body matched antennas for microwave medical imaging are concluded.

6.1. Measurement setup for microwave medical imaging

The measurement setup is constructed for the detection of hemorrhagic stroke. First, the construction of the brain phantom including the realistic dielectric properties is briefly discussed. Based on the shape of the brain phantom, an antenna array is put directly in contact with the brain phantom. After that, the measurement setup of the overall medical diagnosis system is described together with the measurement procedure and data acquisition.

6.1.1. Brain phantom for stroke detection

The demonstrator for stroke detection using microwaves is based on a tissue-simulating phantom, which is a standard norm before a clinical trial is performed. Thus, a brain phantom is required to be constructed for the stroke detection and will be briefly described. Moreover, to better evaluate the improvements of the on-body matched antenna for the medical imaging system without the significant influence of a complicated brain model, the **brain phantom** for the detection of hemorrhagic stroke is simplified to be consisting of the **blood** and an **averaged brain tissue** (averaged permittivity of skull, grey matter and white matter). The goal is to detect the existence and position of the bleeding in the brain. In the following section, a concept of constructing a brain phantom is investigated in terms of its dielectric property and stability. Then, the geometric arrangement of the brain phantom with the blood and averaged brain tissue is provided.

The brain phantom must be constructed to be of a fixed shape according to the realistic scenario. Considering the cost, availability and toxicity, gelatin (bloom 180), sugar and distilled water are chosen to be the ingredients of the phantom. Gelatin helps to fix the shape of the phantom. Sugar and gelatin are soluble in water, which enables a homogeneous mixture. The achieved relative permittivity can be altered by the weight ratio of sugar in the mixture.

The phantom can be produced in three steps: in the first step, the water and sugar are mixed in a pan at room temperature and heated to 60°C. Then, the gelatin is added into the mixture. The mixture must be stirred for it to be homogeneous at around 60°C. In the final step, the mixture is carefully poured into a container (to avoid/remove any air bubbles in the mixture or on the surface) and quickly cooled to 8°C in a refrigerator to avoid any inhomogeneity that might be caused during the cooling process.

Since the measurements with phantom can take a long time and must be repeatable (after a few days), the mixture must be stable with regard to the dielectric properties for a long period. For this purpose, a test phantom (sugar 45%, gelatin 10%, water 45%) was measured three times after different time periods and its dielectric property is plotted in Figure 6.1. It can be observed that a stable dielectric porperty is guaranteed during a period of one week and the conductivity decreases slightly after 3 weeks due to the reduced water content in the mixture. In conclusion, the dielectric property of the phantom based on this concept is very stable for the period of one week. Furthermore, the homogeneity and fixed shape of the whole phantom can be guaranteed.

Based on this concept, the brain phantom including blood and averaged brain tissue can be constructed. The ingredients with weight ratio for the blood and averaged brain tissues, based on the concept discussed before, are provided in Table 6.1 [Gee12].

The shape of the blood and brain phantoms are shown in Figure 6.2. The blood phantom is enclosed within a thin latex bag with a length of 3 cm and radius of 0.5 cm. The averaged brain tissue consists of a cylindrical section (length of 20 cm and radius of 7.5 cm) and a half spherical section as shown in Figure 6.2 (c). The blood phantom is then placed inside the averaged brain tissue. The exact location of the blood phantom will be given later. The presence of the latex between the blood and averaged brain tissue affects the reflection behavior only very slightly thanks to the low thickness of the latex (less than 0.1 mm) compared to the wavelength in the operation frequency range.

Figure 6.3 provides the measured relative permittivities and conductivities of the blood and averaged brain tissue of the constructed phantom. In comparison, the references of the dielectric properties of blood and averaged brain

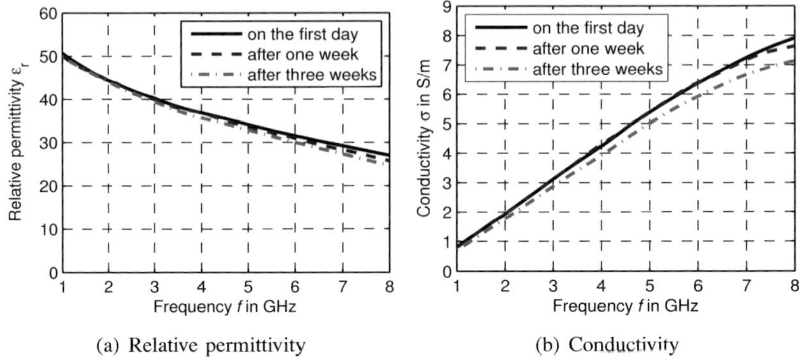

(a) Relative permittivity

(b) Conductivity

Figure 6.1.: Comparison of the relative permittivity (a) and (b) conductivity of the test phantom, measured on the first day, after one week and three weeks.

Table 6.1.: Ingredients of blood and averaged brain tissue for the brain phantom with their weight ratios.

Tissue	Gelatin in %	Sugar in %	Distilled water in %
Blood	11	15	74
Averaged brain tissue	6	47	47

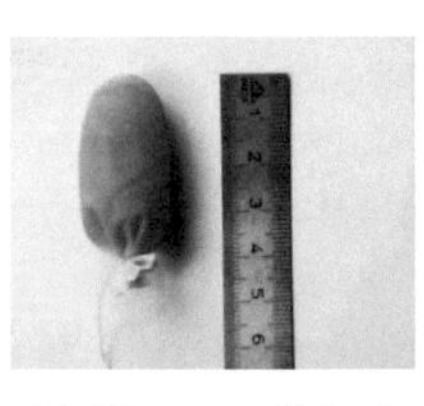

(a) Phantom of blood

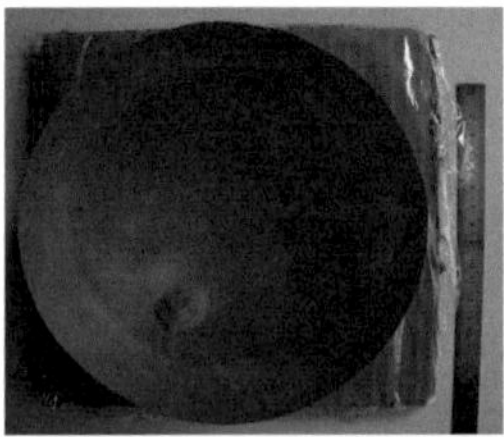

(b) Top view of whole phantom

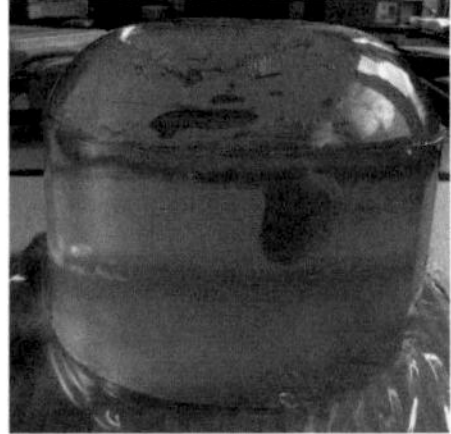

(c) Side view of whole phantom

Figure 6.2.: Photos of the brain phantom for hemorrhagic stroke detection.

tissue according to the Cole-Cole equation are also plotted. The reference of averaged brain tissue is the average of the permittivity of the skin, skull, grey and white matter. Both the relative permittivity and conductivity of the blood phantom agree very well with the reference. The relative permittivity and conductivity of the averaged brain tissue indicate a slight difference compared to its reference. The conductivity of the averaged brain tissue is larger than that of the reference in almost the whole frequency range from 1 to 7 GHz. It increases the signal attenuation and makes the detection more difficult (considered as a worse case). The large difference of the relative permittivity between blood and averaged brain tissue can be clearly seen and can be utilized for the detection of the blood phantom due to the large contrast of the dielectric properties at their boundary.

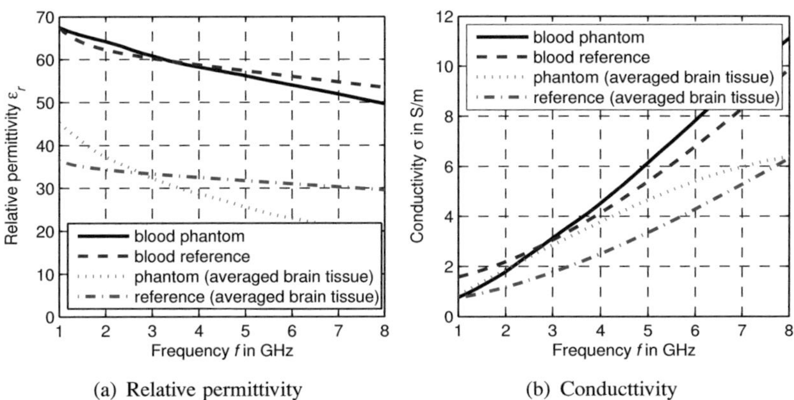

(a) Relative permittivity   (b) Conducttivity

Figure 6.3.: Relative permittivities and conductivities of the blood and averaged brain tissue compared with references from the Cole-Cole equation (averaged permittivity of skull, grey matter and white matter).

To detect the existence and position of the blood within the brain tissue, an antenna array is required to be placed around the phantom to capture the reflections, which will be introduced in the following section.

6.1.2. Array with on-body matched antennas

Since the brain phantom was simplified to be of a nearly cylindrical shape, the antenna elements are arranged in a circular configuration so that each element in the constructed antenna array can be directly in contact with the brain phantom. Moreover, the imaging algorithm can also be simplified, since the captured reflections are based on a circular scan.

To investigate reflections from the target in a wide frequency range in the radar imaging, the differentially-fed slot antennas optimized from 1 to 7 GHz are chosen to construct the antenna array. To allow more antennas to be placed in the circular array, the small-sized stepped-slot antenna with slotline feed network ($26\times35\times36.5\,\mathrm{mm}^3$) is used and an array of 10 antenna elements is constructed as shown in Figure 6.4. Moreover, this antenna exhibits high maximum gain and penetration efficiency at high frequencies compared to the other differentially-fed slot antennas. The shortest dimension of this antenna is 26 mm on the horizontal plane. The main direction of radiation of each antenna points to the center point of the array and the distance between this center point to the surface of the radiator is 75 mm, which corresponds to the radius of the brain phantom. All of the antennas are fixed between two plastic rings with a width of 20 mm and radius of 90 mm.

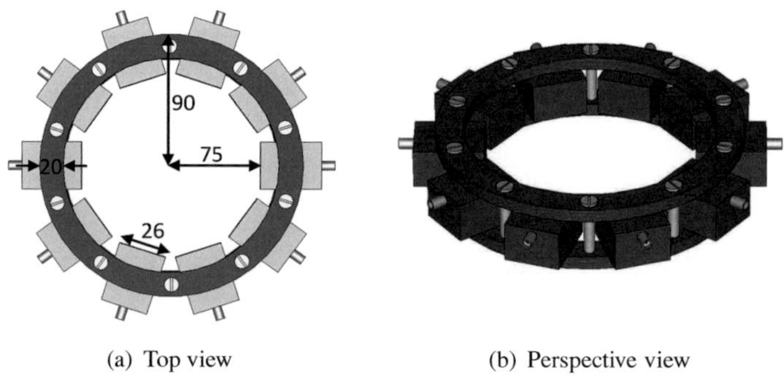

(a) Top view   (b) Perspective view

Figure 6.4.: Array with 10 single antennas in a circular arrangement (unit: mm).

The single antenna configuration is shown in Figure 6.5. To reduce the coupling between adjacent antennas, each antenna is wrapped with absorber material with Styrofoam in between. Vertical polarization is used. The characteristics of the antenna element can be seen in 5.3.4.

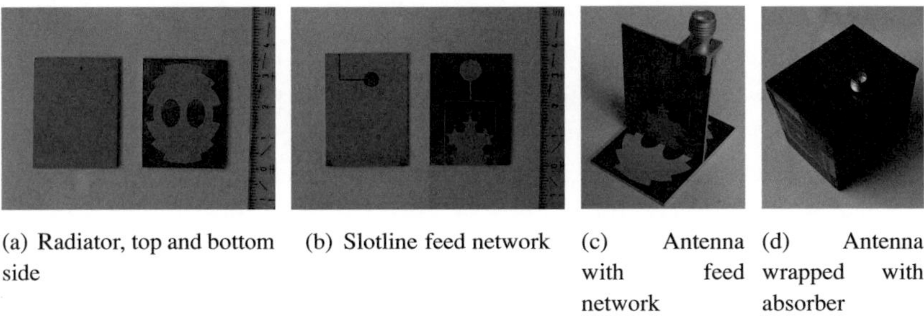

(a) Radiator, top and bottom side

(b) Slotline feed network

(c) Antenna with feed network

(d) Antenna wrapped with absorber

Figure 6.5.: The fabricated stepped-slot antenna with slotline feed network for the construction of the array.

6.1.3. Measurement setup with brain phantom

With the brain phantom and the antenna array, the overall measurement setup for hemorrhagic stroke detection will be introduced.

The frequency sweep approach using a VNA is applied for the medical imaging to achieve a high system dynamic range. The measurement is performed with a frequency sweep from f_{min} to f_{max} in frequency interval of Δf. The transfer function of channel $H_c(f)$ can be obtained from the step-frequency-mode of the VNA. Then the channel impulse response (CIR) $h_c(t)$ in the time domain is obtained through an Inverse Fast Fourier Transformation (IFFT) in (6.1). Furthermore, a window function (Hamming window) with very high side lobe suppression is used before the IFFT to reduce the side lobes in the time domain.

$$h_c(t) = \text{IFFT}(H_c(f)).$$ (6.1)

Though the antennas used are matched in the frequency range from around 1 to 7 GHz, the measured frequency range is set to be from 0.5 to 5 GHz (801 points). It is because the signal attenuation in the brain phantom is too high above 5 GHz and thus the reflections will be too weak to be detected.

The frequency band is divided into many frequency points and a small IF bandwidth is used, which leads to a better SNR. Due to the high SNR, a high measurement accuracy is achievable by using this frequency sweep approach. Otherwise, the decrease of the IF bandwidth increases the whole sweep time and a real time measurement requires large IF bandwidth. Therefore, a compromise between sweep time and SNR must be found for different applications. In the following measurement, an IF bandwidth of 150 Hz is used and the measured time of a whole sweep is in the millisecond range, which is still acceptable for the real time process. The input power of the NWA is set to be 5 dBm and a power amplifier (discussed in 3.2.1) is used.

The overall measurement setup is illustrated in Figure 6.6. The signal is radiated by one antenna (Tx) and the other antennas (Rx) receive the reflections. This is repeated with different antennas as the Tx. With 10 antennas in an array, $10 \times (10 - 1)/2$ unique pairs of antennas and hence 45 signals can be obtained (Tx and Rx are reciprocal). The S_{21} of the VNA is recorded for each transmission pair. For the signal analysis, $S_{i,j}$ is used to denote the measured S_{21} with the ith antenna as Tx and the jth antenna as Rx. In the demonstrator, the response (S_{21}) of the different channels is achieved by manually switching the different antennas.

The signals are recorded for further image processing. For successful image reconstruction, the exact location of each antenna has to be known to determine the corresponding time delay of the useful reflection. Then, based on the recorded data and geometrical arrangement of the antenna array, the microwave image of the detection scenario can be generated using a microwave reconstruction algorithm. With regard to the microwave reconstruction algorithm, a beamforming algorithm will be described in the following sections.

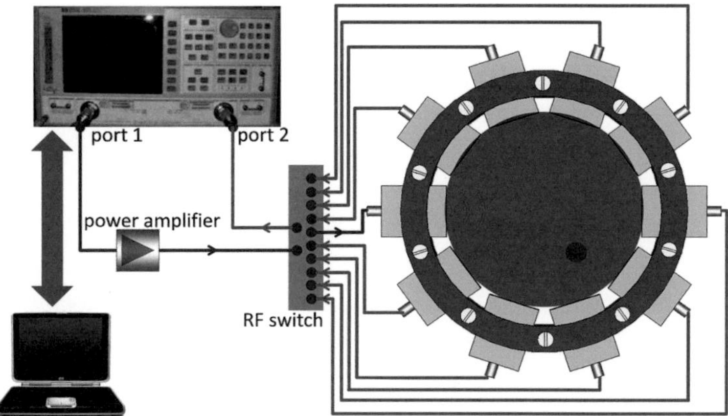

Figure 6.6.: Measurement setup of the medical imaging system for hemorrhagic stroke detection.

6.2. Image reconstruction with beamforming algorithm

For radar imaging, several adaptive/non-adaptive processing approaches have
been developed and applied to wideband medical imaging in the literature.
To obtain a high resolution and low sidelobes of imaging results, an adaptive
technique, which is a time-domain multistatic adaptive microwave imaging
(MAMI), was reported in [XGX+06]. In [OJG10], the data-independent microwave imaging via space-time (MIST) beamforming technique based on
finite impulse response (FIR) filters designed in the frequency domain was
extended and applied to breast cancer detection. The different improvements
of various algorithms will not be discussed further. For the image reconstruction in this thesis, a general beamformer (Delay-and-Sum beamformer)
is used [FLHS02] [19].

Since the proposed antennas are matched directly to the human body, the
strong reflection from the skin in the received signals is inherently eliminated.
However, the recorded signals still contain unwanted responses such as background reflections and antenna coupling, which are of a much higher ampli-

tude than the reflections from the target. Thus, before the imaging reconstruction algorithm is performed, calibration methods to remove unwanted responses are first discussed to enhance the response from the target.

6.2.1. Calibration methods

The goal of the calibration is to remove the residual antenna reverberation, background reflections and strong antenna coupling. Due to the small distance between the antenna elements, a strong direct coupling between Tx and Rx has to be taken into account. The distance between the antenna and the target is also comparable to the space between antennas. Therefore, the antenna coupling cannot be separated and eliminated in the time domain. Moreover, the reflection from the target is very weak due to the high signal attenuation in the brain phantom. Therefore, the useful reflection is overlapped by the antenna coupling, which cannot be separated from the desired reflection. Thus, the antenna coupling has to be calibrated out.

Based on the proposed antenna array, the coupling between different antenna elements in the presence of the brain phantom are measured. The S_{21} of the different channels is measured directly by the NWA. The results are then evaluated in the time domain, where the strongest peak values with regard to the channel impulse response are considered to be the magnitude of the antenna coupling. The coupling between different antenna elements is shown in Figure 6.7. The minimum of the peak is set to be -80 dB, which is located diagonally (no coupling exists for the antenna itself). The results show that the adjacent antennas have the strongest coupling. The antenna coupling decreases significantly with the increasing spacing between the antennas. It has been shown that the antenna coupling is especially dominant when it is adjacent to the Tx. Therefore, the calibration of the antenna coupling is of significant importance for the quality and reliability of the imaging results.

Regarding the aforementioned issue, the reference signal that is the average of the signals from all channels is often used for the calibration. The performance of the averaging calibration is investigated in the following section.

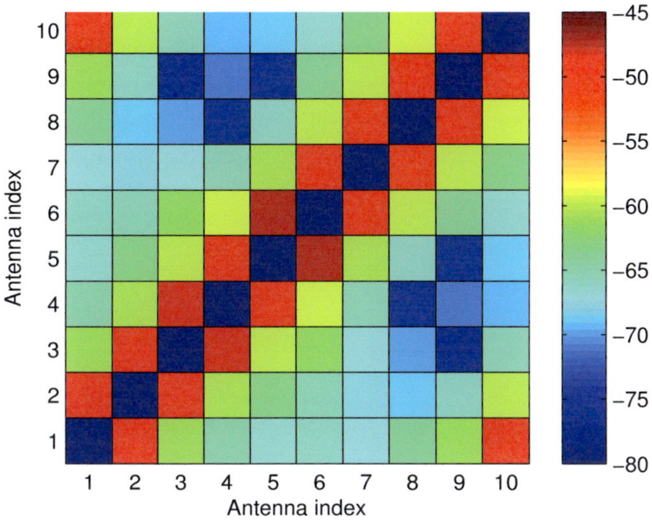

Figure 6.7.: Antenna coupling between different antenna elements of the array (peak value of the CIR in dB).

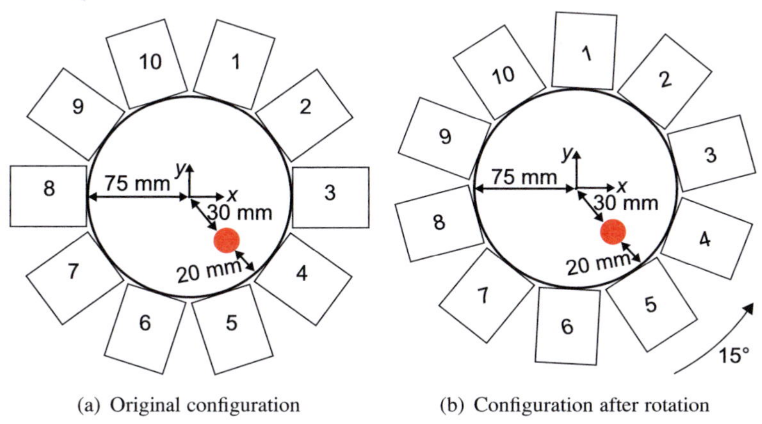

Figure 6.8.: Illustration of the antenna array configuration together with blood phantom before and after rotation.

Averaging calibration

The antenna array configuration with the antenna index and the exact position of the blood phantom is shown in Figure 6.8 (a). The blood phantom is placed in front of antenna 4 and 5 at a distance of around 20 mm. Figure 6.9 shows the photos of the measurement setup of the brain phantom and antenna array.

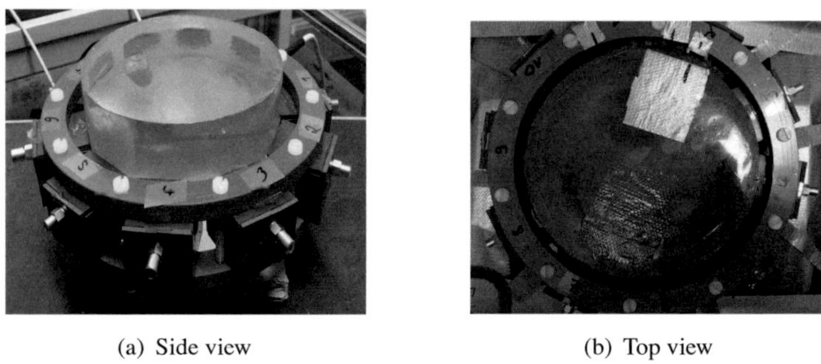

(a) Side view   (b) Top view

Figure 6.9.: Measurement setup with the antenna array and the gelatin phantom.

Before the averaging calibration is performed, the signals $(S_{i,j})$ are transformed into the time domain using the IFFT to obtain $x_{ij}(t)$, which denotes a signal transmitted from the antenna j and received by the antenna i. The signal is measured from 0.5 to 5 GHz and then zero-padding is applied in the frequency domain to increases the time resolution of the signal in the time domain.

The calibration can be mathematically expressed as

$$x_{ij,\text{cal}}(t) \quad = \quad x_{ij}(t) - x_{ij,\text{ref}}(t) \tag{6.2}$$

where $x_{ij,\text{cal}}(t)$ and $x_{ij,\text{ref}}(t)$ are the calibrated and reference signal, respectively.

The reference signal $x_{ij,\text{ref}}(t)$ is generated by averaging all signals separately for the channels with the same space between Tx and Rx, since their coupling is very similar. Therefore, 5 different groups of reference signals are needed for the calibration of all signals (0, 1, 2, 3 or 4 antennas between Tx and Rx).

156

After that the reference signals for 5 groups are obtained, each signal $x_{ij}(t)$ is subtracted by its reference signal.

In comparison, a rotation calibration will be introduced in the following section.

Rotation calibration

The calibrated signal using rotation calibration can be written as

$$x_{ij,\text{cal}}(t) \;=\; x_{ij}(t) - x_{ij,\text{rot}}(t), \tag{6.3}$$

where $x_{ij,\text{rot}}(t)$ are the recorded reference signals after rotation.

For the rotation calibration, the overall array is rotated $15°$ anti-clockwise around the center point of the array as shown in Figure 6.8 (b). Altogether two measurements must be performed based on the original arrangement (original signals $x_{ij}(t)$) and the arrangement after the rotation (reference signals $x_{ij,\text{rot}}(t)$). For each channel, the background reflection and antenna coupling are calibrated with its reference signal (the same transmission pair after rotation). Since the antennas and antenna distance remain the same, the background reflection and antenna coupling can be successfully calibrated. Otherwise, the response from the target changes slightly with array arrangement before and after rotation in terms of time delay and amplitude and hence the calibrated signal still represents the response from the target.

Though the rotation calibration requires two measurements, the antenna coupling can be completely calibrated, since the reference signal is obtained for each channel, respectively.

6.2.2. Delay and Sum beamformer

The Delay and Sum (DAS) beamformer [FLHS02] is a passive process, in which the backscattered signals are first assigned with appropriate time delays so that the beamformer focuses on a specific point inside the target region. Afterwards the time-aligned signals are added and the energy of the resulting signal which corresponds to the intensity level of a focal point within the imaging area is estimated. In this thesis, the DAS beamformer is based on the time domain signals, which are obtained from the wideband measured data in the frequency domain (using IFFT).

Considering that the signal radiated from the Tx (antenna index i), propagates to the target, the response from the target can be received by the Rx (antenna index j) (i and j could be any single antenna of the array), the output of a DAS beamformer is given by:

$$y(t) = \sum_{j=i+1}^{N} \sum_{i=1}^{N} w_{ij} x_{ij}(t - \tau_{ij}) = \sum_{j=i+1}^{N} \sum_{i=1}^{N} w_{ij} x_{ij}(t - \frac{d_{ij}}{c_m}), \qquad (6.4)$$

where τ_{ij} is the time delay of the propagation, which is determined by the total distance d_{ij} from Tx to target and from target to Rx with regard to the propagation velocity of the waves in medium c_m. Including τ_{ij} in the beamforming, the different time delays are then compensated and hence the signals can be coherently added to reconstruct the target as shown in Figure 6.10.

w_{ij} is the beamformer apodization weights (window function), which is of significance for the optimization of the shape of the peak and the suppression of the sidelobes of the signals. A Hamming window is also used in the beamformer.

The DAS beamformer described above has several benefits and drawbacks. From (6.4), it can be observed that the DAS beamformer is carried out on each received signal independently. Moreover, the DAS beamformer features simplicity and robustness of the signal processing. However, its performance is limited in terms of the artifact removal and the resolution of the image [19]. To improve the artifact removal effect and the resolution of the image, a coherence factor (CF) is introduced. The coherence factor coefficients are defined as the ratio of the coherent sum of the signals and the non-coherent sum of the signals. This can be written as

$$CF(t) = \frac{2 \left| \sum_{j=i+1}^{N} \sum_{i=1}^{N} x_{ij}(t - \tau_{ij}) \right|^2}{N(N-1) \sum_{j=i+1}^{N} \sum_{i=1}^{N} \left| x_{ij}(t - \tau_{ij}) \right|^2}. \qquad (6.5)$$

The CF coefficients are multiplied directly to the output signal $y(t)$ of the DAS beamformer. By taking these coefficients into account, the directivity of

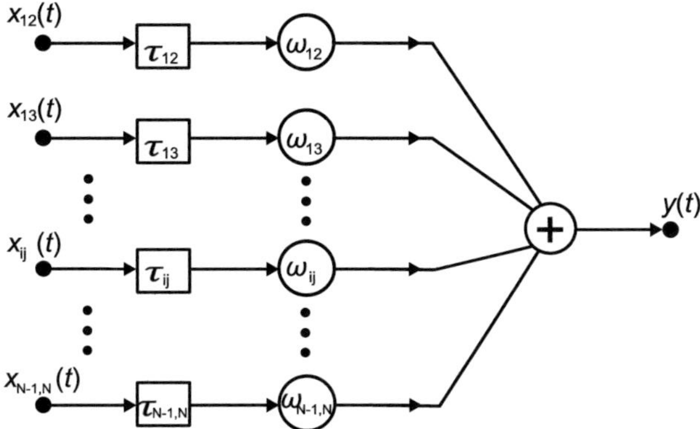

Figure 6.10.: Block diagram of the Delay-and-Sum beamformer.

the beamformer can be considerably increased, which increases the dynamic range of the imaging result and improves significantly the resolution of the microwave image.

6.3. Analysis of calibrated signals and 2D imaging results

Having the DAS beamforming in mind, the calibrated signals obtained from the measured data as well as the processed two-dimensional (2D) microwave images will be analyzed and discussed in terms of dynamic range of image (range of peak level and noise level of the image), signal-to-clutter ratio (SCR) and image resolution.

Figure 6.11 shows the received signal from the adjacent antennas (antenna index 1, 2, 3, 4 and 5) based on the configuration in Figure 6.8 (a). The antenna coupling is dominant before the calibration is performed. In the signals after calibration using the averaging method, the reflection from the blood phantom can be clearly identified especially in x_{45}. Therefore, with very careful measurements, the reflection from the target (blood phantom) is visible in the time domain. The strongest reflection occurs around at $t = 3.6$ ns.

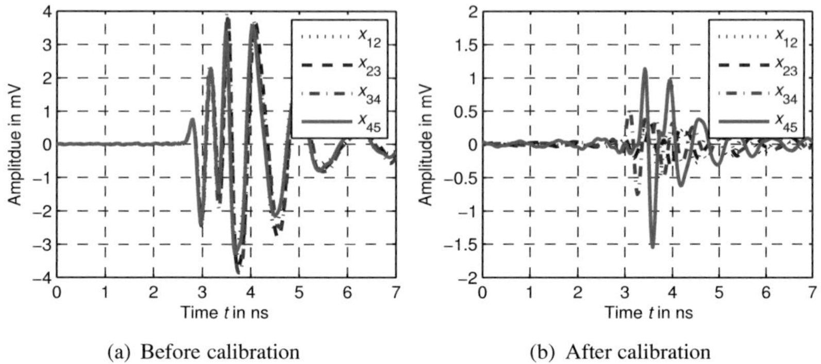

(a) Before calibration   (b) After calibration

Figure 6.11.: Received signals before and after averaging calibration of the channels of adjacent antennas (antenna index: 1, 2, 3, 4, and 5) in the time domain.

The width of the pulse refers to the signal bandwidth, which is determined by the bandwidth of the antennas. Weak ringing effects can also be observed, which are caused by the non-linearity of the antenna and additional multi-reflections in the phantom. Using these results in the time domain, the signals are processed using the beamforming algorithm.

The processed microwave image (xy-plane refer to Figure 6.8) is shown in Figure 6.12(a). For a better comparison with the real setup, the microwave image together with the antenna array is shown in Figure 6.12(b). The position of the blood can be clearly identified, which agrees with the real location of the blood in the brain phantom. However, different clutters are also visible in the microwave image and can be regarded as ghost targets caused by the averaging calibration. A very strong reflection is observed in the calibrated x_{78} in the time domain, which results in the strong clutter in the image in front of antenna 7 and 8.

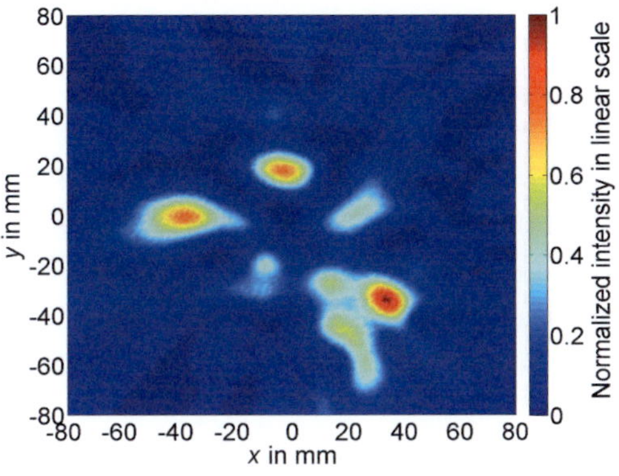

(a) Processed microwave image

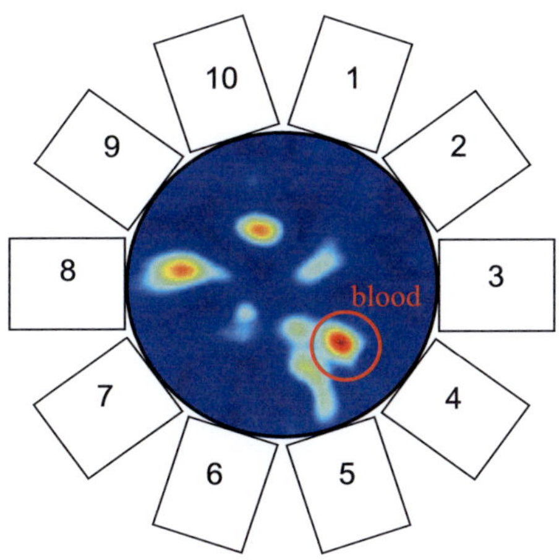

(b) Processed microwave image together with antenna array

Figure 6.12.: Processed microwave image using DAS-algorithm (averaging calibration).

From the imaging result (see Figure 6.12(a)), it can be observed that the averaging calibration has a low SCR level, since strong clutter signals are caused by the nonideal calibration.

To perform a better calibration of the background reflection and antenna coupling, the rotation calibration is introduced based on an additional measurement with a rotation ($15°$) of the antenna array (see Figure 6.8 (b)). The calibrated signals of some channels in Figure 6.13 using rotation calibration show that reflections in x_{57} and x_{58} contribute to the final imaging results.

The processed microwave image with the rotation calibration is shown in Figure 6.14(a). A strong reflection is observed at ($x = 2\,\text{cm}$, $y = -3.5\,\text{cm}$), which is estimated to be the blood phantom. The blood phantom appears in the image with better contrast and its position is estimated with good accuracy compared to the result using averaging calibration. The image together with the array configuration in Figure 6.14(b) demonstrates that the blood phantom is clearly represented in the right location in the brain phantom. Otherwise, some weak clutters are still identified. The SCR of the image is estimated to be $6\,\text{dB}$, which allows the detection of the target (the blood).

It can be seen that the SCR of the processed image using the rotation calibration is improved significantly, compared to the result using averaging calibration. The image result indicates also lower sensitivity to the position error of the antennas between measured signals and reference signals.

The benefit of the averaging calibration procedure is that only one measurement is required compared to the rotation calibration. However, it must be assumed that the signals recorded from different channels in the same group exhibit similar background reflection and antenna coupling. In practice, however, this cannot be achieved and a slight difference of the coupling between adjacent antennas introduces clutter after calibration, which results in the inaccuracy of this calibration method. The reason for the different coupling is that the fabricated antennas cannot feature exactly the same impedance matching and radiation properties. On the other hand, a not 100% uniform arrangement of the antenna in a circular configuration also causes inaccuracy of the antenna position and slight differences of the antenna spacing. This results in different antenna coupling in the same group and hence the difference is averaged and included in each reference signal. Due to this dif-

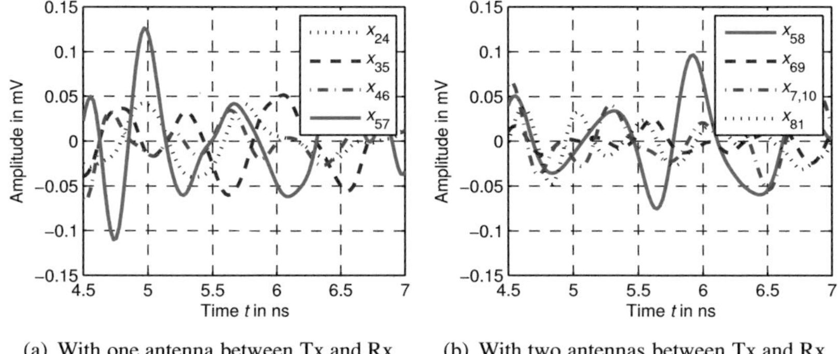

(a) With one antenna between Tx and Rx   (b) With two antennas between Tx and Rx

Figure 6.13.: Received signals calibrated with rotation calibration in the time domain.

ference, ghost reflections are caused in the calibrated signal and cannot be distinguished from the realistic reflections. To reduce this effect, the antennas should be fabricated very carefully to assure almost the same performance and the antennas should be placed uniformly.

Due to the better performance of the rotation calibration, this calibration method will be used for further investigation of the microwave imaging system.

To demonstrate the influence of the signal bandwidth on the microwave image, the bandwidth of the received signals using the rotation calibration are limited to 2.5 GHz (0.5-3 GHz). From the processed imaging result in Figure 6.15, the degradation of the imaging result in terms of SCR and resolution can be clearly identified. This result confirms that the contribution of higher frequencies (between 3 to 5 GHz) to the imaging result is significant, though the signal attenuation in lossy medium (brain phantom) at the higher frequencies is considerably higher compared to lower frequencies. Therefore, the designed on-body matched antennas must feature, besides very low operational frequency, a large operational bandwidth, which has been discussed in chapter 5.

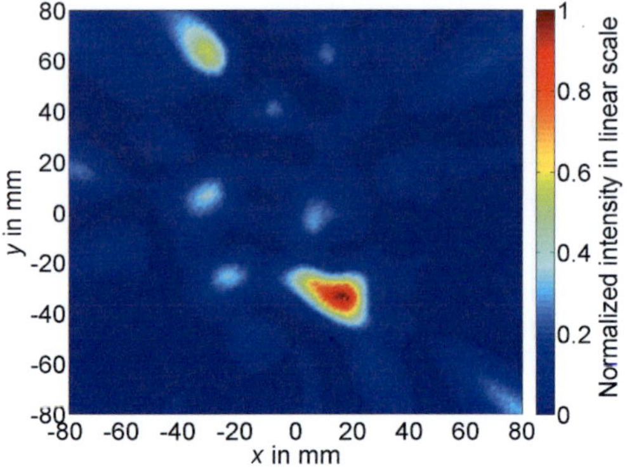

(a) Processed microwave image

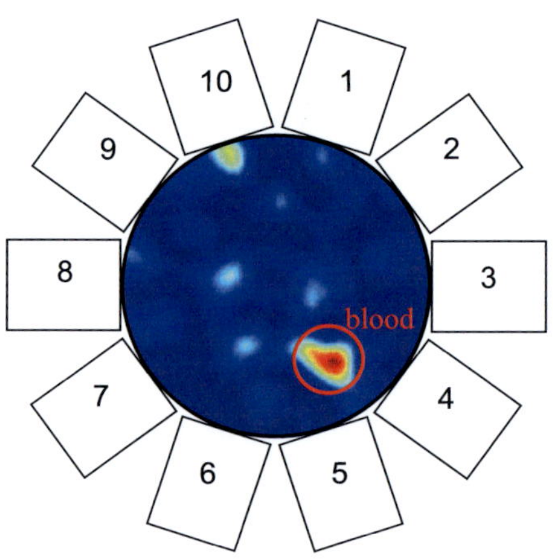

(b) Processed microwave image together with antenna array

Figure 6.14.: Processed microwave image together with antenna array (rotation calibration).

For microwave medical imaging, a large number of antennas in an array are desirable to obtain more scattered information from the target. The effect of the number of antennas on the imaging result is investigated based on the received signals using the rotation calibration. To compare the imaging result with 10 antennas, only 5 antennas (antenna index 1, 3, 5, 7, and 9 based on the configuration in Figure 6.8) are now used to transmit or receive signals and $5\times(5\text{-}1)/2{=}10$ signals are available for the imaging algorithm. The imaging result (see Figure 6.16) shows that the SCR is strongly degraded and the clutters are stronger than the response from the target. It can be seen that the large number of antennas in the array is of significance to the detection capability of the microwave medical imaging system. This confirms that the on-body matched antennas are required to be miniaturized. It is due to the fact that the small-sized antennas enable a large number of antennas to be arranged in an array within a limited space for the scenario in medical diagnosis. In this way, more reflections from the target can be captured by the antenna array. Since the antennas are required to have very low operational frequency, the miniaturization of the on-body matched antennas (discussed in chapter 5) becomes more challenging due to the increased wavelength.

In terms of dynamic range of the processed images, the values based on the mentioned different procedures (calibration method, frequency range and number of used antennas) are summarized in Table 6.2. A slightly higher dynamic range is achieved using averaged calibration, since the signals are averaged and hence the noise level is suppressed. The three procedures based on rotation calibration have only slight differences in terms of dynamic range of the processed images. The results agrees with the analysis that the dynamic range is strongly dependent on the used radar approach in terms of signal modulations (PN, IR-UWB, frequency sweep approach) and the transmitted power.

6.3.1. Summary

A feasibility study of the detection of the human hemorrhagic stroke using microwave imaging is provided, which is based on an on-body matched antenna array characterized from 1 to 7 GHz and a brain phantom (consisting averaged brain tissue and blood phantom). In the image processing, the DAS

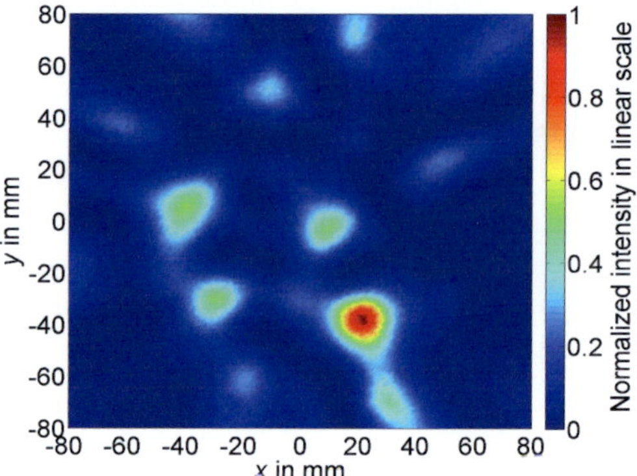

Figure 6.15.: Microwave image processed by DAS-algorithm: rotation calibration, reduced bandwidth effect (frequency range from 0.5 and 3 GHz).

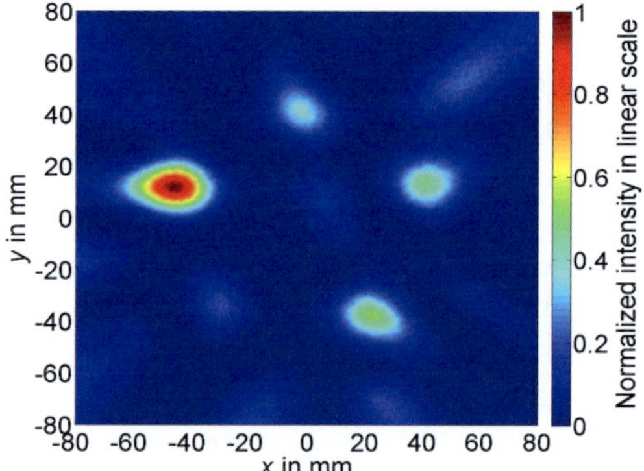

Figure 6.16.: Microwave image processed by DAS-algorithm: rotation calibration, reduced antenna elements in the array (5 antennas in the array used).

Beamformer is applied to reconstruct the target in the measurement scenario. From the imaging results, it has to be emphasized that the blood phantom is

Table 6.2.: The dynamic range of the images based on different process procedures.

Process procedure	Antenna number	Frequency range	Dynamic range
Averaging calibration	10	0.5 to 5 GHz	36 dB
Rotation calibration	10	0.5 to 5 GHz	31 dB
Rotation calibration	5	0.5 to 5 GHz	29.1 dB
Rotation calibration	10	0.5 to 3 GHz	28.7 dB

successfully reconstructed in the right location in the image compared to the imaging results with the antennas in free space, in which the detection was only feasible in the simulation and no promising results can be verified in the measurement [20] [Riv11]. The reason is that, in case of the off-body antenna, the antenna coupling and the strong reflection from the air-skin boundary as well as the impedance mismatching of the antennas caused by placing them closely to the phantom, degrade the received signals. The useful reflections cannot be reconstructed using the calibration method. Therefore, it is of significance to match the antennas to the human body (phantom), since the signal level of reflection is strongly improved benefiting from the elimination of the reflection from the air-skin boundary as well as the achieved good impedance matching of the antennas in contact with the human body.

It has been shown that small-sized antennas with a stable phase front improved the location accuracy in the DAS beamformer. This is because the operational range is comparable to the antenna size. Thus, the determination of the phase front of the antenna is of significance for the image processing. The small size and the stable phase front over frequency help to obtain a correct delay time of the received signals. Moreover, a significant improvement of the microwave images is achieved in terms of SCR and contrast by increasing the number of antenna elements in the array. The clutter in the image with 10 antennas was suppressed compared to the result with 5 antennas. Therefore, the miniaturization of the single antenna contributes considerably to the microwave imaging in terms of enabling more antenna elements to be used within a limited space.

The bandwidth of the antenna also strongly affects the image quality. The wideband operation using the proposed on-body matched antenna enables the wideband medical imaging, in which significant improvements in resolution and artifact reduction have been achieved. It can be further emphasized that even better image resolution and SCR can be achieved by optimizing the imaging algorithm. However, further improvement of the algorithm is not within the framework of this thesis.

The successful detection of the blood phantom embedded in averaged brain tissue confirmed the applicability of the on-body matched antenna for the microwave medical imaging. The recorded signals by the on-body matched antennas feature high SNR and contain more useful information than that of antenna matched in free space.

7. Summary and conclusions

In this thesis, new concepts of body-matched antennas for microwave medical applications were developed, where the antennas are directly in contact with the human body or implanted in the human body. The antenna designs serve mainly to conduct microwave medical diagnosis and data telemetry. Therefore, two categories of antennas were designed for microwave medical diagnosis (on-body matched antennas) and data telemetry (implantable antennas). With these, a new future telemedicine home system can be envisioned, in which the vital signs of the patients can be monitored in real time and hence their mobility as well as their quality of life can be improved. Concepts were developed with antenna miniaturization techniques to result in a compact size for the intended medical devices and to maintain the high radiation performance in terms of the impedance matching, efficiency and radiation pattern. Application-wise, a high directivity and front-to-back ratio are desirable for the on-body matched antennas for medical diagnosis, while an omni-directional pattern is required for implantable antennas. With these challenges in mind, the contributions of each chapter are summarized in the following paragraphs.

Chapter 2 provided a preliminary study for the design of the body-matched antennas. Through the quantitative investigation of human tissues in terms of dielectric properties, the propagation behavior of EM-waves in human tissues was evaluated from the system point of view. Based on the high dielectric contrast between the target (tumor, urine, etc.) and surrounding tissues, the reflection from their boundaries can be detected for diagnostic purposes. The results showed that a very high system dynamic range is required to capture the reflected weak signal. With regard to the operational frequency range, the lower frequencies enable a high penetration into the human body and the large frequency range contributes to a higher bandwidth and hence a finer range resolution. Depending on the applications (diagnosis with wideband signal or data telemetry with narrow band signal) and location of sensors in the human body, an optimal operational frequency can be arranged in the consideration of the SNR of the system and the radiation regulations. Furthermore, with this knowledge, the design requirements and specifications of on-body matched and implantable antennas have been specified for microwave medical systems.

In chapter 3, characterization methods were introduced to evaluate the performance of body-matched antennas. For the verification, two antenna measurement systems with tissue-simulating liquid for the characterization of body-matched antennas are provided, whose characterization of the radiation cannot be performed in an anechoic chamber due to the presence of the lossy human body. The E-field probe based measurement system allows the direct measurement of the antenna pattern at a short distance (40-60 mm), while the planar near-field system is designed to obtain the far-field antenna pattern by applying the NF-FF transformation. High measurement accuracy can be assured by the use of a precise positioning system with a high precision stepper motor. Such antenna measurement systems allow the validation of the simulation results of on-body matched and implantable antennas with respect to the impedance matching, near-field and far-field pattern.

The body-matched antenna designs for data transmission of IMDs and diagnosis are provided respectively in chapter 4 and 5. All of the antennas are matched to different human tissues depending on the location of the devices and optimized together with the tissue model for the highest performance with respect to impedance matching, radiation efficiency and radiation pattern. Miniaturization techniques contribute significantly to the reduction of the antenna size. Furthermore, the design was focused on optimizing the antenna structure and the current distribution at different frequencies.

In chapter 4, three stripline-fed implantable slot antennas at the ISM band were designed. The antennas have an omni-directional pattern especially in the H-plane, that allows a robust wireless connection between implants and external devices, independent of the location and orientation of the patients to the base station. Based on optimization of the antenna structure, the antenna (M3-3) was miniaturized to a size of $10.45 \times 12.9\,\mathrm{mm}^2$, with a size reduction of more than 40% compared to the original one (M3-1), allowing a significant size reduction of the IMDs. Due to the stripline-fed configuration and good impedance matching (under -10 dB) in muscle tissues, the implantable antenna features a high radiation efficiency (94.2%) and gain (4.3 dBi), which enable data telemetry between implants and external devices with high efficiency.

For medical diagnosis, different on-body matched antennas operating at different frequency bands were proposed in chapter 5. By matching the antennas directly to the human skin, very high front-to-back ratio of the radiation pattern is achieved, which significantly improves the SNR of the antenna system. The small-sized differentially-fed slot antenna characterized from 1 to 7 GHz enables the construction of a microwave medical imaging system with high resolution for the detection of e.g. breast cancer. To achieve deeper penetration of the microwave signals into the human body, a dual-band slotted Bowtie antenna and a wideband folded double-layer Bowtie antenna were designed. By applying a folded structure and meandered microstrip lines at the bottom of the Bowtie antenna, a small size of $30 \times 30\,mm^2$ with a size reduction of 40% is achieved, compared to the reference antenna (regular Bowtie antenna at $50 \times 50\,mm^2$). These antennas can either be used in radar-based imaging or tomography. The small-sized antennas with the lowest operational frequency of 0.5 GHz, high radiation efficiency, high front-to-back ratio and relatively high gain improve the penetration depth and the SNR of received signals, which showed a high potential for microwave medical diagnosis.

In chapter 6, the applicability of the on-body matched antenna for medical diagnosis was confirmed. The measurement demonstrator using a tissue-simulating phantom and an array of 10 stepped slot antennas show the high detection capability for stroke thanks to the low operational frequency, high front-to-back ratio and small antenna size. The blood phantom was successfully detected with good SCR, although very weak reflected signals were received due to a strong signal attenuation in the brain phantom during the propagation. Without the aforementioned features, the off-body antenna cannot detect the weak reflection. The results confirmed that the on-body matched antenna significantly improved the SNR of the reflections compared to the off-body antenna. Furthermore, the small-sized differentially-fed slot antenna allows for a large number of elements for the array in a limited space, which also improves the image quality with respect to the resolution and SCR. It has been confirmed that the miniaturization techniques, which have been applied to the body-matched antenna design, contributed very positively to the performance of the microwave medical imaging.

In conclusion, the following considerable contributions of this thesis can be emphasized:

- The quantitative investigation of the wave propagation in human tissues was studied, which allows the specification of the required antennas in terms of the lowest operational frequency, bandwidth, directivity and etc, depending on the applications and the location on/in the human body.

- For the first time in the literature, two antenna measurement systems were developed, which facilitate the validation of both near-field and far-field patterns of the on-body matched and implantable antennas immersed in a tissue-simulating liquid.

- Miniaturization techniques of the antennas based on extending the electrical length and regulating the current flow in the antenna structure at different frequencies were developed. Multiband resonances, independent surface current regulation at lower and higher frequencies for wideband antenna as well as fractal structure for miniaturization also for suppression of unwanted radiation are proposed, by which significant size reductions of the antenna operated at 1 GHz and even 0.5 GHz were achieved.

- Design methods (such as introducing slotted ground, stripline-feed and aperture-coupling) for the prevention of radiation loss caused by surface and leaky waves due to the surrounded lossy tissues. High radiation efficiency and a stable pattern have been achieved.

- The applicability of the on-body matched antennas is successfully verified with a microwave imaging system for the detection of hemorrhagic stroke, where a deep penetration of the microwaves are required.

The proposed design principles of the various antennas as well as the miniaturization techniques can be extended to the general design of antennas for medical applications in the presence of the human body, or even for antennas in free space. The achieved small-sized antennas at different frequency bands contribute directly to compact medical sensors (i.g. portable sensors for diagnosis or IMDs). Moreover, the promising results of the detection of hemorrhagic stroke using a simplified brain phantom with the proposed antenna array encouraged further research to be conducted including the use of even lower frequencies for high penetration ability and advanced imaging algorithms. All these contributions enable an extension of the medical applications using microwaves with the objective to obtain more advanced healthcare systems.

A. Parameters of tissues based on Cole-Cole equation

Tissue	ε_∞	$\Delta\varepsilon_1$	$\tau_1(\mathrm{ps})$	α_1	$\Delta\varepsilon_2$	$\tau_2(\mathrm{ns})$	α_2
muscle	4.0	50.0	7.23	0.10	7000	353.6	0.10
skin	4.0	39.0	7.96	0.10	280	79.58	0.00
w. matter	36.71	0.29	8.04	0.24	-	-	-
g. matter	55	0.5	7.76	0.12	-	-	-
blood	4.0	56.0	8.38	0.10	5200	132.6	0.10
bone	2.5	18.0	13.26	0.22	300	79.58	0.25
fat	2.5	3.0	7.96	0.20	15	15.92	0.10
skull	2.5	10.0	13.26	0.22	180	79.58	0.20

Tissue	$\Delta\varepsilon_3$	$\tau_3(\mu\mathrm{s})$	α_3	$\Delta\varepsilon_4$	$\tau_4(\mathrm{ms})$	α_4	σ
muscle	1.2×10^6	318.31	0.10	2.5×10^7	2.274	0.00	0.20
skin	3.0×10^4	1.59	0.16	3.0×10^4	1.592	0.20	0.0004
w. matter	-	-	-	-	-	-	0.47
g. matter	-	-	-	-	-	-	1.03
blood	0.0			0.0			0.70
bone	2.0×10^4	159.15	0.20	2.0×10^7	15.91	0.00	0.70
fat	3.3×10^4	159.15	0.05	1.0×10^7	7.958	0.01	0.01
skull	5.0×10^3	159.15	0.20	1.0×10^5	15.91	0.00	0.20

Table A.1.: Parameters of Cole-Cole equation used to predict the dielectric properties of different tissues.

Bibliography

[ABWZ09]   G. Adamiuk, S. Beer, W. Wiesbeck, and T. Zwick. Dual-Orthogonal Polarized Antenna for UWB-IR Technology. *IEEE Antennas and Wireless Propagation Letters*, 8:981–984, 2009.

[Ada10]   G. Adamiuk. *Methoden zur Realisierung von dual-orthogonal, linear polarisierten Antennen für die UWB-Technik.* Phd thesis, Karlsruher Institut für Technologie (KIT), Karlsruhe, 2010.

[AKS13]   S. Ashok Kumar and T. Shanmuganantham. Implantable CPW Fed Circular Slot Antenna for ISM Band. In *National Conference on Communications (NCC)*, Feburary 2013.

[ARNT11]   R. K. Amineh, M. Ravan, N. K. Nikolova, and A. K. Tpour. Three-Dimensional Near-Field Microwave Holography Using Reflected and Transmitted Signals. *IEEE Transactions on Antennas and Propagation*, 59(12):4777–4789, December 2011.

[ARTN11]   R. K. Amineh, M. Ravan, A. Trehan, and N. K. Nikolova. Near-Field Microwave Imaging Based on Aperture Raster Scanning with TEM Horn Antennas. *IEEE Transactions on Antennas and Propagation*, 59(3):928–940, March 2011.

[Bal05]   C. A. Balanis. *Antenna Theory: Analysis and Design.* Wiley-Interscience, New York, 3rd edition, 2005.

[Bar12]   A. Barouni. Weiterentwicklung einer am Körper angepassten UWB-Antenne für die Schlaganfalldiagnostik. Bachelor thesis, Institut für Hochfrequenztechnik und Elektronik, Karlsruher Institut für Technologie (KIT), Karlsruhe, November 2012.

[BBH70]   T. W. Barber, J. A. Brockway, and L. S. Higgins. The Density of Tissues in and about the Head. *Acta Neurologica Scandinavica*, 46(1):85–92, March 1970.

[BLM06]   D. Baudry, A. Louis, and B. Mazari. Characterization of the Open Ended Coaxial Probe Used for Near-Field Measurements in EMC Applications. *PIER, Progr. Electromagn. Res.*, 60:311–333, 2006.

[BSAG$^+$00]   S. Boyer, M. Sawan, M. Abdel-Gawad, S. Robin, and M. M. Elhilali. Implantable Selective Stimulator to Improve Bladder Voiding: Design and Chronic Experiments in Dogs. *IEEE Transactions on Rehabilitation Engineering*, 8(4):464–470, December 2000.

[CBHVV04]   M. Converse, E. J. Bond, S. C. Hagness, and B. D. Van Veen. Ultrawide-Band Microwave Space-Time Beamforming for Hyperthermia Treatment of Breast Cancer: A Computational Feasibility Study. *IEEE Transactions on Microwave Theory and Techniques*, 52(8):1876–1889, August 2004.

[CKK04]   A. Christ, A. Klingenböck, and N. Kuster. Exposition durch Körpernahe Sender im Rumpfbereich, Arbeitspaket I: Bestandsaufnahme. Foundation for Research on Information Technologies in Society, Swiss Federal of Technology - ETHZ, December 2004.

[CLC95]   CENELEC CLC/TC111B. Human Exposure to Electromagnetic Fields: High Frequency (10 KHz to 300 GHz). Technical report, European Prestandard (pr ENV 50166-2), Brussels, 1995.

[Com01]   Federal Communications Commission. Evaluating Compliance with FCC Guidelines for Human Exposure to Radiofrequency Electromagnetic Fields. Supplement C to OET Bulletin 65, June 2001.

[dCHS$^+$11] F. S. di Clemente, M. Helbig, J. Sachs, U. Schwarz, R. Stephan, and M. A. Hein. Permittivity-Matched Compact Ceramic Ultra-Wideband Horn Antennas for Biomedical Diagnostics. In *5th European Conference on Antennas and Propagation (EUCAP)*, April 2011.

[Deb60] P. Debye. *Polar Molecules*. Dover Publications, New York, 1960.

[DFG$^+$08] F. D'Agostino, F. Ferrara, C. Gennarelli, R. Guerriero, and M. Migliozzi. An Effective NF-FF Transformation Technique with Planar Spiral Scanning Tailored for Quasi-Planar Antennas. *IEEE Transactions on Antennas and Propagation*, 56(9):2981–2987, Sepember 2008.

[ESSK00] T. Endo, Y. Sunahara, S. Satoh, and T. Katagi. Resonant Frequency and Radiation Efficiency of Meander Line Antennas. *Electronics and Communications in Japan (Part II: Electronics)*, 83(1):52–58, January 2000.

[FAB$^+$07] J. Ferlay, P. Autier, M. Boniol, M. Heanue, M. Colombet, and P. Boyle. Estimates of the Cancer Incidence and Mortality in Europe in 2006. *Ann Oncol.*, 18(3):581–92, 2007.

[FCC02] *Revision of Part 15 of the Commission's Rule Regarding Ultra-Wideband Transmission Systems.* First Report and Order, Federal Communications Commision (FCC), Februar 2002.

[FG95] J. Fromm, R. E. Varon and L. R. Gibbs. Congestive Heart Failure and Pulmonary Edema for the Emergency Physician. *Journal of Emergency Medicine*, 13(1):71–87, 1995.

[FLHS02] E. C. Fear, X. Li, S. C. Hagness, and M. A. Stuchly. Confocal Microwave Imaging for Breast Cancer Detection: Localization of Tumors in Three Dimensions. *IEEE Transactions on Biomedical Engineering*, 49(8):812–822, August 2002.

[Gee12]   D. Geenen. Aufbau und Optimierung eines körperangepassten UWB-Antennenarrays für die Schlaganfalldiagnostik. Bachelor thesis, Institut für Hochfrequenztechnik und Elektronik, Karlsruher Institut für Technologie (KIT), October 2012.

[GGC96]   C. Gabriel, S. Gabriel, and E. Corthout. The Dielectric Properties of Biological Tissues: I. Literature Survey. *Phys. Med. Biol.*, 41(11):2231–2249, November 1996.

[GJR10]   M. Guardiola, L. Jofre, and J. Romeu. 3D UWB Tomography for Medical Imaging Applications. In *IEEE Antennas and Propagation Society International Symposium (AP-SURSI)*, July 2010.

[GLG96a]   S. Gabriel, R. W. Lau, and C. Gabriel. The Dielectric Properties of Biological Tissues: II. Measurements in the Frequency Range 10 Hz to 20 GHz. *Phys. Med. Biol.*, 41(11):2251–2269, November 1996.

[GLG96b]   S. Gabriel, R. W. Lau, and C. Gabriel. The Dielectric Properties of Biological Tissues: III. Parametric Models for the Dielectric Spectrum of Tissues. *Phys. Med. Biol.*, 41(11):2271–2293, November 1996.

[GMP07]   S. F. Gregson, J. McCormick, and C. Parini. *Principles of Planar Near-Field Antenna Measurements*. Institution of Engineering and Technology, 2007.

[GMZ$^+$10]   C. Gilmore, P. Mojabi, A. Zakaria, M. Ostadrahimi, C. Kaye, S. Noghanian, L. Shafai, S. Pistorius, and J. LoVetri. A Wideband Microwave Tomography System with a Novel Frequency Selection Procedure. *IEEE Transactions on Biomedical Engineering*, 57(4):894–904, April 2010.

[Guy84]   A. W. Guy. History of Biological Effects and Medical Applications of Microwave Energy. *IEEE Transactions on Microwave Theory and Techniques*, 32(9):1182–1200, September 1984.

[HLC$^+$11] F. Huang, C. Lee, C. Chang, L. Chen, T. Yo, and C. Luo. Rectenna Application of Miniaturized Implantable Antenna Design for Triple-Band Biotelemetry Communication. *IEEE Transactions on Antennas and Propagation*, 59(7):2646–2653, July 2011.

[Hol38]   H. E. Hollmann. *Das Problem der Behandlung biologischer Körper im Ultrakurz-Wellen-Strahlungsfeld*. G. Thieme, Leipzig, 1938.

[Hur85]   W. D. Hurt. Multiterm Debye Dispersion Relations for Permittivity of Muscle. *IEEE Transactions on Biomedical Engineering*, BME-32(1):60–64, January 1985.

[ITU01]   Sharing between the Meteorological Aids Service and Medical Implant Communications Systems (MICS) Operating in the Mobile Service in the Frequency Band 401-406 MHz. International Telecommunications Union Recommendation (ITU-R) Std. ITU-R Recommendation SA 1346, 2001.

[Kap96]   D. S. Kapp. Efficacy of Adjuvant Hyperthermia in the Treatment of Superficial Recurrent Breast Cancer: Confirmation and Future Directions. *Int. J. Rad. Oncol. Biol. Phys.*, 35:117–1121, 1996.

[Kar04]   A. Karlsson. Physical Limitations of Antennas in a Lossy Medium. *IEEE Transactions on Antennas and Propagation*, 52(8):2027–2033, August 2004.

[KCL$^+$09] M. Klemm, I. J. Craddock, J. A. Leendertz, A. Preece, and R. Benjamin. Radar-Based Breast Cancer Detection

Using a Hemispherical Antenna Array - Experimental Results. *IEEE Transactions on Antennas and Propagation*, 57(6):1692–1704, July 2009.

[KGA$^+$09]   D. D. Krishna, M. Gopikrishna, C. K. Aanandan, P. Mohanan, and K. Vasudevan. Compact Wideband Koch Fractal Printed Slot Antenna. *IET Microwaves, Antennas & Propagation*, 3(5):782–789, August 2009.

[KHT08]   T. Karacolak, A. Z. Hood, and E. Topsakal. Design of a Dual-Band Implantable Antenna and Development of Skin Mimicking Gels for Continuous Glucose Monitoring. *IEEE Transactions on Microwave Theory and Techniques*, 56(4):1001–1008, April 2008.

[KKYP01]   J. Kim, K. Kim, J. Yook, and H. Park. Compact Stripline-fed Meander Slot Antenna. *Electronics Letters*, 37(16):995–996, August 2001.

[KRS04]   J. Kim and Y. Rahmat-Samii. Implanted Antennas Inside a Human Body: Simulations, Designs, and Characterizations. *IEEE Transactions on Microwave Theory and Techniques*, 52(8):1934–1943, August 2004.

[KRS06]   J. Kim and Y. Rahmat-Samii. Planar Inverted-F Antennas on Implantable Medical Devices: Meandered Type versus Spiral Type. *Microwave and Optical Technology Letters*, 48(3):567–572, March 2006.

[Lan09]   N. Langendorf. Ischemic & Hemorrhagic Stroke Report. Technical report, Center for Health Information Analysis, 2009.

[LBVVH05]   X. Li, E. J. Bond, B. D. Van Veen, and S. C. Hagness. An Overview of Ultra-Wideband Microwave Imaging via Space-Time Beamforming for Early-Stage Breast-Cancer Detection. *IEEE Antennas and Propagation Magazine*, 47(1):19–34, February 2005.

[LHC93]   H. J. Liebe, G. A. Hufford, and M. G. Cotton. Propagation Modelling of Moist Air and Suspended Water/Ice Particles at Frequencies below 1000 GHz. In *AGARD 52nd Special Meeting of the Panel on Electromagnetic Wave Propagation, Adv. Group for Aerosp. Res. and Dev.*, Palmade Mallorca, May 1993.

[LS94]   D. Lamensdorf and L. Susman. Baseband-Pulse-Antenna Techniques. *IEEE Antennas and Propagation Magazine*, 36(1), February 1994.

[MBZ^{+}11]   F. Merli, L. Bolomey, J. Zurcher, G. Corradini, E. Meurville, and A. K. Skrivervik. Design, Realization and Measurements of a Miniature Antenna for Implantable Wireless Communication Systems. *IEEE Transactions on Antennas and Propagation*, 59(10):3544–3555, October 2011.

[MD99]   G. H. Markx and C. L. Davey. The Dielectric Properties of Biological Cells at Radiofrequencies: Applications in Biotechnology. *Enzyme and Microbial Technology*, 25(3-5):161–171, August 1999.

[MJ13]   J. Ma and A. Jemal. *Breast Cancer Metastasis and Drug Resistance*. Springer, New York, 1st edition, 2013.

[Moo63]   R. Moore. Effects of a Surrounding Conducting Medium on Antenna Analysis. *IEEE Transactions on Antennas and Propagation*, 11(3):216–225, May 1963.

[MV98]   S. M. Metev and V. P. Veiko. *Laser Assisted Microtechnology*. Springer, Berlin, Germany, 2nd edition, 1998.

[Nik11]   N. K. Nikolova. Microwave Imaging for Breast Cancer. *IEEE Microwave Magazine*, 12(7):78–94, December 2011.

[NMdS^{+}07]   A. Natarajan, M. Motani, B. de Silva, K. K. Yap, and K. C. Chua. Investigating Network Architectures for Body Sensor Networks. In *HealthNet 2007*, June 2007.

[OJG10]   M. O'Halloran, E. Jones, and M. Glavin. Quasi-Multistatic MIST Beamforming for the Early Detection of Breast Cancer. *IEEE Transactions on Biomedical Engineering*, 57(4):pp.830–840, April 2010.

[oNiRPI98] International Commission on Non-ionizing Radiation Protection (ICNIRP). ICNIRP Guidelines for Limiting Exposure to Time-varying Electric, Magnetic and Electromagnetic Fields (up to 300 GHz). *Health Physics*, 74(4):494–522, April 1998.

[Poz]   D. M. Pozar. *Microwave Engineering*. Hoboken: Wiley, 3rd edition.

[QLD03]   H. Qian, P. C. Loizou, and M. F. Dorman. Phone-Assistive Devices Based on Bluetooth Technology for Cochlear Implant Users. *IEEE Transactions on Neural Systems Rehabilitation Engineering*, 11(3):282–287, 2003.

[Rei98]   J. P. Reilly. *Applied Bioelectricity: From Electrical Stimulation to Electropathology*. Springer, 1998.

[RFFea07]   W. Rosamond, K. Flegal, G. Friday, and et al. Heart Disease and Stroke Statistics-2007 Update: a Report from the American Heart Association Statistics Committee and Stroke Statistics Subcommittee. *Circulation*, 115(5):69–171, 2007.

[Riv11]   J. Rivera. UWB-Imaging-System zur Detektion von Wasseransammlungen im menschlichen Körper. Diploma thesis, Institut für Hochfrequenztechnik und Elektronik, Karlsruher Institut für Technologie (KIT), January 2011.

[Roe99]   R. B. Roemer. Engineering Aspects of Hyperthermia Therapy. *Annual Review of Biomedical Engineering*, 1:347–376, 1999.

[Sam12]   K. Chu Sam. Aufbau eines Messsystems zur Charakterisierung von an Gewebe angepassten Antennen. Bachelor thesis, Institut für Hochfrequenztechnik und Elektronik,

Karlsruher Institute für Technologie (KIT), Karlsruhe, March 2012.

[Sch10]   S. Scherr.   UWB-Pseudo-Noise-Radaruntersuchungen für medizinische Anwendungen.   Diploma thesis, Institut für Hochfrequenztechnik und Elektronik, Karlsruher Institut für Technologie (KIT), Karlsruhe, October 2010.

[SCK07]   G. Shobha, R. R. Chittal, and K. Kumar. Medical Applications of Wireless Networks. In *Second International Conference on Systems and Networks Communications (ICSNC)*, August 2007.

[SDMS05]   C. J. Simon, D. E. Dupuy, and W. W. Mayo-Smith. Microwave Ablation: Principles and Applications. *Radiographics*, 25:69–83, October 2005.

[Ser09]   Medical Device Radiocommunications Service. Federal Communication Commission Std. CFR, Part 95.601-673 Subpart E, Part 95.1201-1221 subpart I, 2009.

[SFC04]   P. Soontornpipit, C. M. Furse, and You Chung Chung. Design of Implantable Microstrip Antenna for Communication with Medical Implants. *IEEE Transactions on Microwave Theory and Techniques*, 52(8):1944–1951, August 2004.

[Shu88]   B. Shuppert. Microstrip/Slotline Transitions: Modeling and Experimental Investigation. *IEEE Transactions on Microwave Theory and Techniques*, 36(8):1272–1282, August 1988.

[SKR+11]   M. L. Scarpello, D. Kurup, H. Rogier, D. Vande Ginste, F. Axisa, J. Vanfleteren, W. Joseph, L. Martens, and G. Vermeeren. Design of an Implantable Slot Dipole Conformal Flexible Antenna for Biomedical Applications. *IEEE Transactions on Antennas and Propagation*, 59(10):3556–3564, October 2011.

[Smi75]   Glenn S. Smith. A Comparison of Electrically Short Bare and Insulated Probes for Measuring the Local Radio Frequency

Electric Field in Biological Systems. *IEEE Transactions on Biomedical Engineering*, BME-22(6):477–483, November 1975.

[SSC94] B. M. Steinhaus, R. E. Smith, and P. Crosby. The Role of Telecommunications in Future Implantable Device Systems. In *the 16th Annual International Conference of the IEEE Engineering in Medicine and Biology Society*, Baltimore, 1994.

[Ste23] H.E. Stewart. *Diathermy and Its Application to Pneumonia*. P. B. Hoeber, inc., 1923.

[SW05] W. Sörgel and W. Wiesbeck. Influence of the Antennas on the Ultra-Wideband Transmission. *EURASIP Journal on Applied Signal Processing*, 2005:296–305, January 2005.

[TDGL11] K. F. Tong, A. Dufour, L. Ge, and K. M. Luk. Beamscanning Probe Antennas for Deep Brain Stimulation. In *Proceedings of the 5th European Conference on Antennas and Propagation (EUCAP)*, Rom, April 2011.

[TP08] H. Trefna and M. Persson. Antenna Array Design for Brain Monitoring. In *Antennas and Propagation Society International Symposium AP-S*, San Diego, July 2008.

[TRVdVG95] T. N. Tulasidas, G. S. V. Raghavan, F. Van de Voort, and R. Girard. Dielectric Properties of Grapes and Sugar Solutions at 2.45 GHz. *Journal of the Microwave Power and Electromagnetic Energy*, 33(2):117–123, 1995.

[USNLoM] National Institutes of Health United States National Library of Medicine. The Visible Human Project MRI Scans.

[Vat10] E. Vatamaniuc. UWB-Systemkonzeptuntersuchungen zur Detektion von Wasseransammlungen im menschlichen Körper. Diploma thesis, Institut für Hochfrequenztechnik und Elektronik, Karlsruher Institut für Technologie (KIT), 2010.

[VC09]   L. Venkatraghavan and V. Chinnapa. Non-Cardiac Implantable Electrical Devices: Brief Review and Implications for Anesthesiologists. *Can. J. Anesth.*, 56:320–326, 2009.

[VRK06]   A. Vander Vorst, A. Rosen, and Y. Kotsuka. *RF/Microwave Interaction with Biological Tissues*. Wiley-IEEE Press, 2006.

[WDJ$^+$96] J. A. Warren, R. D. Dreher, R. V. Jaworski, J. J. Putzke, and R. J. Russie. Implantable Cardioverter Defibrillators. *Proceedings of the IEEE*, 84(3):468–479, March 1996.

[WSTI09]   X. Wei, K. Saito, M. Takahashi, and K. Ito. Performances of an Implanted Cavity Slot Antenna Embedded in the Human Arm. *IEEE Transactions on Antennas and Propagation*, 57(4):894–899, April 2009.

[XGX$^+$06] Y. Xie, B. Guo, L. Xu, J. Li, and P. Stoica. Multistatic Adaptive Microwave Imaging for Early Breast Cancer Detection. *IEEE Transactions on Biomedical Engineering*, 53(8):1647–1657, August 2006.

[Yan11]   J. Yan. Entwurf und Charakterisierung von UWB-Antennen zur Abstrahlung in den menschlichen Körper für medizinische Diagnostik. Bachelor thesis, Institut für Hochfrequenztechnik und Elektronik, Karlsruher Institut für Technologie (KIT), Karlsruhe, November 2011.

[You12]   W. You. Development of a Miniaturized Antenna for Wireless Communication of Implantable Sensors. Bachelor thesis, Institut für Hochfrequenztechnik und Elektronik, Karlsruher Institut für Technologie (KIT), Karlsruhe, November 2012.

[ZL07]   K. Zhang and D. Li. *Electromagnetic Theory for Microwaves and Optoelectronics*. Springer, Tsinghua University, Beijing, 2nd edition, 2007.

Own publications

Journal publications

[1] X. Li, G. Adamiuk, E. Pancera, and T. Zwick. Physics-Based Propagation Characterisations of UWB Signals for the Urine Detection in Human Bladder. *Int. J. Ultra Wideband Communications and Systems*, 2(2):94–103, December 2011.

[2] X. Li, M. Jalilvand, Y. L. Sit, and T. Zwick. A Compact Double-Layer On-Body Matched Bowtie Antenna for Medical Diagnostics. *IEEE Transactions on Antennas and Propagation (accepted)*, 2013.

[3] X. Li, Y. L. Sit, L. Zwirello, and T. Zwick. A Miniaturized UWB Stepped-Slot Antenna for Medical Diagnostic Imaging. *Microwave and Optical Technology Letters*, 55(1):105–109, January 2013.

Conference publications

[4] X. Li, M. Janson, G. Adamiuk, C. Heine, and T. Zwick. A 2D Ultra-Wideband Indoor Imaging System with Dual-Orthogonal Polarized Antenna Array. In *COST 2100*, Athens, February 2009.

[5] J. Schmid, E. Pancera, X. Li, L. Niestoruk, S. Lamparth, W. Stork, and T. Zwick. Ultra-Wideband Detection System for Water Accumulations in the Human Body. In *11 th International Congress of the IUPESM-Medical Physics and Biomedical Engineering World Congress - WC2009*, Munich, Germany, September 2009.

[6] H. Wu, X. Li, and T. Zwick. Motion Compensation of Automotive SAR for Parking Lot Detection,. In *International Radar Symposium (IRS)*, Hamburg, September 2009.

[7] X. Li, G. Adamiuk, M. Janson, and T. Zwick. Polarization Diversity in Ultra-Wideband Imaging Systems. In *International Conference on Ultra Wideband- ICUWB 2010*, Nanjing, September 2010.

[8] X. Li, E. Pancera, L. Zwirello, H. Wu, and T. Zwick. Detection of Water Accumulation in the Human Bladder with Ultra Wideband Radar. In *COST 2100*, Athens, February 2010.

[9] X. Li, E. Pancera, L. Zwirello, H. Wu, and T. Zwick. Ultra Wideband Radar for Water Detection in the Human Body. In *German Microwave Conference GeMiC*, Berlin, March 2010.

[10] E. Pancera, X. Li, T. Zwick, and W. Wiesbeck. Fidelity Criterion for UWB Medical Diagnostic. In *IEEE International Conference on Ultra-Wideband*, Nanjing, September 2010.

[11] E. Pancera, X. Li, T. Zwick, and W. Wiesbeck. UWB Antennas for Medical Diagnostics Purposes. In *IEEE Antennas and Propagation Society International Symposium*, Toronto, Juli 2010.

[12] E. Pancera, X. Li, L. Zwirello, and T. Zwick. Performance of Ultra Wideband Antennas for Monitoring Water Accumulation in Human Bodies. In *European Conference on Antennas and Propagation*, Barcelona, April 2010.

[13] J. Schmid, E. Pancera, L. Niestoruk, X. Li, S. Lamparth, T. Zwick, and W. Stork. Ultra-Wideband Signals for the Detection of Water Accumulations in the Human Body. In *International Conference on Bio-inspired Systems and Signal Processing BIOSIGNALS*, Valencia, January 2010.

[14] H. Wu, X. Li, and T. Zwick. Motion Compensation for Landmine Detecting Vehicle-borne SAR. In *International Radar Symposium (IRS)*, Vilnius, June 2010.

[15] L. Zwirello, E. Pancera, X. Li, and T. Zwick. Ultra-Wideband Localization Systems - Possibilities, Challenges and Solutions. In *COST ic0803*, Lausanne, Switzerland, November 2010.

[16] G. Adamiuk, C. Rusch, X. Li, M. Janson, and T. Zwick. Dual-Polarized UWB Antenna for High-Resolution-Imaging-Systems. In *IEEE International Workshop on Antenna Technology (iWAT)*, Hong Kong, March 2011.

[17] M. Jalilvand, X. Li, T. Zwick, W. Wiesbeck, and E. Pancera. Hemorrhagic Stroke Detection Via UWB Medical Imaging. In *Europan Conference on Antennas and Propagation EuCAP*, Rome, April 2011.

[18] M. Jalilvand, X. Li, T. Zwick, W. Wiesbeck, and E. Pancera. UWB SAR Medical Imaging via Broadband Minimum Distortionless Response MVDR Algorithm. In *Europan Conference on Antennas and Propagation (EuCAP)*, Rome, April 2011.

[19] M. Jalilvand, E. Pancera, X. Li, T. Zwick, and W. Wiesbeck. A Sparse Synthetic-Aperture Based UWB Medical Imaging System. In *German Microwave Conference (GeMiC)*, Darmstasdt, March 2011.

[20] X. Li, M. Jalilvand, L. Zwirello, and T. Zwick. Array Configurations of a UWB Near Field Imaging System for the Detection of Water Accumulation in Human Body. In *the European Radar Conference (EuRAD)*, Manchester, October 2011.

[21] X. Li, M. Jalilvand, L. Zwirello, and T. Zwick. Synthetic Aperture-Based UWB Imaging System for Detection of Urine Accumulation in Human Bladder. In *IEEE International conference on Ultra Wideband (ICUWB)*, Bologna, September 2011.

[22] X. Li, S. Scherr, L. Sit, E. Pancera, and T. Zwick. Performance Analysis of Various UWB Radar Approaches for Medical Diagnostics. In *Proceedings of the IEEE International Microwave Symposium*, Baltimore, USA, June 2011.

[23] X. Li, S. Scherr, H. Wu, E. Pancera, and T. Zwick. Feasibility Study of an Ultra Wideband Pseudo-Noise-Radar for Medical Applications. In *Proceedings of the IEEE European Conference on Antennas and Propagation*, Rom, Italy, April 2011.

[24] E. Pancera, H. Barba, X. Li, M. Jalilvand, and T. Zwick. Uwb antennas optimization for in-body radiation. In *German Microwave Conference (GeMiC)*, Darmstadt, Germany, March 2011.

[25] E. Pancera, X. Li, M. Jalilvand, T. Zwick, and W. Wiesbeck. Uwb medical diagnostic: In-body transmission modeling and applications. In *European Conference on Antennas and Propagation (EuCAP)*, Rom, April 2011.

[26] J. Pontes, G. Adamiuk, S. Beer, L. Zwirello, X. Li, and T. Zwick. Novel Design Method for Frequency Agile Beam Scanning Antenna Arrays. In *IEEE International Workshop on Antenna Technology (iWAT)*, 2011.

[27] S. Scherr, X. Li, S. Ayhan, and T. Zwick. A Polarity Correlator in a UWB-PN-Radar for the Detection of Multiple Targets. In *European Radar Conference (EuRAD)*, Manchester, October 2011.

[28] H. Wu, L. Zwirello, X. Li, L. Reichardt, and T. Zwick. Motion Compensation with One-axis Gyroscope and Two-axis Accelerometer for Automotive SAR. In *German Microwave Conference GeMiC*, Darmstadt, March 2011.

[29] L. Zwirello, X. Li, E. Pancera, and T. Zwick. An Ultra-Wideband Communication System with Localization Capabilities - Hardware Realization of HF-Frontend Modules. In *6th Management Comitee/Working Group Meeting and Workshop COSTic0803*, Perugia, Italy, April 2011.

[30] M. Jalilvand, X. Li, and T. Zwick. Improved Minimum Variance Processing for UWB Medical Imaging Applications. In *European Radar Conference*, Amsterdam, October 2012.

[31] X. Li, M. Jalilvand, J. Yan, and T. Zwick. Compact Double-Elliptical Slot-Antenna for Medical Applications. In *IEEE European Conference on Antennas and Propagation*, Prague, March 2012.

[32] X. Li, K. Chu Sam, W. Wiesbeck, and T. Zwick. A Planar Near-Field Measurement System of UWB Antennas for Medical Diagnostics. In *International Conference on Electromagnetics in Advanced Applications*, Cape Town, September 2012.

[33] X. Li, Y. L. Sit, L. Zwirello, M. Jalilvand, and T. Zwick. An E-Field Probe Based Near-Field Measurement System for On- and In-Body Antennas. In *European Microwave Conference (EuMC)*, Amsterdam, October 2012.

[34] X. Li, L. Zwirello, M. Jalilvand, and T. Zwick. Design and Near-field Characterization of a Planar On-body UWB Slot-Antenna for Stroke Detection. In *IEEE International Workshop on Antenna Technology (iWAT)*, Tucson, USA, March 2012.

[35] L. Zwirello, C. Heine, X. Li, T. Schipper, and T. Zwick. SNR Performance Verification of Different UWB Receiver Architectures. In *European Microwave Conference (EuMC)*, Amsterdam, October 2012.

[36] L. Zwirello, L. Reichardt, X. Li, and T. Zwick. Impact of the Antenna Impulse Response on Accuracy of Impulse-Based Localization Systems. In *6th European Conference on Antennas and Propagation*, Prague, March 2012.

[37] M. Jalilvand, X. Li, and T. Zwick. A Model Approach to the Analytical Analysis of Stroke Detection using UWB Radar. In *Europan Conference on Antennas and Propagation (EuCAP)*, Gothenburg, April 2013.

[38] M. Jalilvand, X. Li, L. Zwirello, and T. Zwick. Sensititvity Analysis of UWB Minimum Variance Beamformer for Medical Imaging. In *European Microwave Conference*, Nuernberg, Germany, October 2013.

[39] X. Li, M. Jalilvand, W. You, W. Wiesbeck, and T. Zwick. An Implantable Stripline-Fed Slot Antenna for Biomedical Applications. In *IET International Radar Conference*, Xi An, April 2013.

[40] X. Li, W. Wiesbeck, and T. Zwick. Design considerations for UWB antennas. In *7th European Conference on Antennas and Propagation (EuCAP)*, Gothenburg, April 2013.

[41] Y. L. Sit, X. Li, L. Reichardt, H. Liu, R. Liu, and T. Zwick. A Planar Dual-mode UWB Antenna for an Indoor MIMO Communication System. In *International Workshop on Antenna Technology (iWAT)*, Karlsruhe, Germany, March 2013.

[42] Y. L. Sit, L. Reichardt, X. Li, H. Liu, R. Liu, and T. Zwick. Dual-Orthogonal Mode Planar Antenna for Indoor UWB MIMO Communication Systems. In *IEEE International Symposium on Antennas and Propagation (IEEE-APS)*, Orlando Florida, USA, July 2013.